SELF-ASSESS

CLINICAL PHA

HENRY L. ELLIOTT
MD, MRCP
Senior Lecturer in Clinical Pharmacology

in association with

JOHN L. REID
DM, FRCP
Regius Professor of Materia Medica

PETER C. RUBIN
DM, MRCP
Wellcome Trust Senior Fellow

BRIAN WHITING
MD, FRCP
Professor of Clinical Pharmacology

All of the Department of Materia Medica
University of Glasgow

BLACKWELL SCIENTIFIC PUBLICATIONS
OXFORD LONDON EDINBURGH
BOSTON PALO ALTO MELBOURNE

© 1987 by Blackwell Scientific
Publications Editorial offices:
Osney Mead, Oxford, OX2 0EL
8 John Street, London, WC1N 2ES
23 Ainslie Place, Edinburgh, EH3 6AJ
52 Beacon Street, Boston,
  Massachusetts 02108, USA
667 Lytton Avenue, Palo Alto,
  California 94301, USA
107 Barry Street, Carlton, Victoria 3053,
  Australia

First published 1987

Set by Holmes McDougall Ltd,
Edinburgh, and printed and bound by
Billings and Sons Limited, London,
Oxford, and Worcester.

DISTRIBUTORS

USA
  Year Book Medical Publishers
  35 East Wacker Drive
  Chicago, Illinois 60601

Canada
  The C.V. Mosby Company
  5240 Finch Avenue East,
  Scarborough, Ontario

Australia
  Blackwell Scientific Publications
    (Australia) Pty Ltd
  107 Barry Street
  Carlton, Victoria 3053

**British Library
Cataloguing in Publication Data**

Elliott, Henry L.
  Self-assessment in clinical
  pharmacology.
  1. Chemotherapy——Examinations,
  questions, etc.
  I. Title
  615.5'8'076   RM262

ISBN 0-632-01395-8

Contents

Preface

This volume on *Self-Assessment in Clinical Pharmacology* complements *Lecture Notes on Clinical Pharmacology,* 2nd Edition (Reid J. L., Rubin P. C. & Whiting B., Blackwell Scientific Publications, Oxford) and provides undergraduates and postgraduates with a means of assessing their general understanding of the subject. While it should prove useful as an aid to revision and preparation for examinations, the questions and answers are also designed to be a test of knowledge and a source of explanation and clarification. It is obviously not a comprehensive and detailed examination of all aspects of clinical pharmacology, but has been based on the questions which have been set in recent years in multiple choice examinations for third and fourth year medical students at the University of Glasgow.

Self-Assessment in Clinical Pharmacology consists of standard multichoice questions, comprising an initial 'stem' followed by five statements to create five individual questions, each of which requires a 'true' or 'false' answer. Any number may be correct. Section I is designed to test the reader's knowledge of basic principles and fundamental concepts and accordingly the questions are arranged in subsections relating to a particular topic, e.g. cardiovascular pharmacology, antimicrobial drugs, etc. The answers are given at the end of each subsection.

The questions in Section II are randomly arranged and are directed towards indications and contraindications, adverse effects and particular points about drug usage.

Section III is organized with a different format and is oriented towards therapeutic and clinical practice. Four MCQs (i.e. 20 individual questions) are set to test knowledge covering a case study. Clinically relevant information is given and augmented, and each MCQ addresses a problem as the case is developed.

In both Sections II and III the answers are given on the reverse of the questions.

Although the principal objective of this book is to help the reader acquire and consolidate a knowledge of clinical pharmacology, it should also encourage a grounding in good therapeutic practice and promote an awareness of the risks and benefits associated with drug treatment.

Glasgow, June 1986   Henry Elliott, John Reid,
                                                          Peter Rubin, Brian Whiting

Acknowledgements

We are very grateful to many colleagues and friends who helped to review the questions and answers.

We are grateful to Miss Eleanor Newell for her considerable help in typing the manuscript and collating the questions and answers in this book.

We have tried to ensure that there are no mistakes in the text or answers. There may still be ambiguous questions and instances where acceptable alternative answers could be given. We accept responsibility for any such mistakes or misunderstandings and would be glad to hear of any major disagreements or differences of opinion.

SECTION I

Clinical Pharmacology
Questions

1 Systemic bioavailability:
(a) Is calculated from a comparison of the areas under the plasma concentration–time curves after intravenous and oral administration.
(b) Is always less than 100% following intravenous administration.
(c) Is high for drugs which undergo extensive first-pass hepatic metabolism.
(d) Is often different if the drug is taken fasting instead of with food.
(e) May be altered by the pharmaceutical formulation.

2 First-order kinetics
(a) Implies that the rate of drug metabolism is proportional to drug concentration.
(b) Is more common than zero-order kinetics at concentrations encountered in clinical practice.
(c) Is described by exponential processes.
(d) May not always be exhibited by phenytoin at therapeutic concentrations.
(e) Implies a direct proportionality between dose rate and steady-state concentration.

3 Following an intravenous dose of 100 mg, a drug which shows first-order elimination from a one-compartment model has a plasma half-life of eight hours:
(a) 50 mg will be cleared in eight hours.
(b) 25 mg will be cleared in four hours.
(c) 75 mg will be cleared in 16 hours.
(d) If an oral dose of 100 mg is administered instead, 50 mg will still be eliminated in eight hours.
(e) The plasma concentration will fall to 1/8 original concentration after 24 hours.

4 A one-compartment model implies that:
(a) The decreasing plasma concentration of a drug with time is described by a single exponential term.
(b) A single exponential term may describe the rise in plasma concentration following oral administration.
(c) The drug does not penetrate tissues.
(d) The drug is restricted to the intravascular compartment.
(e) The drug is highly protein-bound.

5   Drugs which are highly lipid-soluble:
(a)   Do not usually penetrate the central nervous system.
(b)   Have high apparent volumes of distribution.
(c)   Are readily absorbed from the gastrointestinal tract.
(d)   Are readily excreted by the kidney without prior metabolism.
(e)   Generally have very long elimination half-lives.

6   Drug binding to plasma proteins:
(a)   Is increased in chronic renal failure.
(b)   Usually involves plasma albumin.
(c)   In the case of lignocaine is largely dependent on alpha$_1$ acid glycoprotein.   + prazosin
(d)   Is more than 90% for warfarin.
(e)   If extensive, is usually associated with a high apparent volume of distribution.

7   Enzyme induction by carbamazepine means that:
(a)   More drug-metabolizing enzyme is present in the liver.
(b)   A more active type of enzyme is present in the liver.
(c)   The efficacy of concurrent oral contraceptive drugs can be compromised.
(d)   The bioavailability of concurrent sodium valproate will be increased.
(e)   The dose of carbamazepine itself often has to be increased.

8   Hepatic drug-metabolizing capacity may be increased by:
(a)   Alcoholism.
(b)   Hepatic cirrhosis.
(c)   Thyrotoxicosis.
(d)   Cardiac failure.
(e)   Untreated epilepsy.

9   When considering pharmacokinetics:
(a)   The peak plasma concentration is directly dependent on the patient's liver or kidney function.
(b)   The volume of distribution denotes the circulating blood volume.
(c)   The elimination half-life is likely to be prolonged if there is liver or kidney failure.
(d)   The volume of distribution for a given drug may vary according to factors such as sex, height, weight and degree of obesity.
(e)   The higher the concentration of a drug, the faster is its rate of subsequent decline.

10 **Which of the following would you expect from a lipid-soluble drug?**
   (a) Likely to appear in the saliva.
   (b) Poor oral absorption.
   (c) Crosses placenta easily.
   (d) Greater likelihood of toxicity in liver disease.
   (e) Reduced excretion in renal failure.

Clinical Pharmacology
Answers

1 (a) *True.* It is the ratio of the AUC following oral administration to the AUC following intravenous administration: it is most commonly expressed as a percentage.

(b) *False.* It is 100% for a drug which is directly administered into the systemic circulation.

(c) *False.* Because of first-pass metabolism, typically in the liver, relatively little drug reaches the systemic circulation.

(d) *True.* Food, and other drugs, may interfere with the process of absorption and occasionally may also influence the rate and extent of metabolism.

(e) *True.* The extent of absorption of a drug may vary considerably as a result of changes in formulation.

2 (a) *True.* With first-order kinetics the rate of the reaction (which may be absorption, distribution, metabolism, elimination) is directly proportional to the concentration or amount of drug present. Thus, the rate increases as the concentration increases, and vice versa. This is usually expressed by the exponential equation:

$$C_t = C_0 e^{-kt}$$

where C_t = concentration of the reactant at time t
C_0 = initial reactant concentration
k = the rate constant (of the reaction).

(b) *True.* With zero-order kinetics the rate of the reaction is fixed (constant). This is uncommon in clinical pharmacology. It occurs when enzyme processes are saturated. Both alcohol and phenytoin demonstrate zero-order kinetics.

(c) *True.* The equation, $C_t = C_0 e^{-kt}$, is typical of exponential equations which describe first-order processes.

(d) *False.* With phenytoin, enzyme saturation occurs with concentrations as low as 10–20 mg/l, leading to zero-order kinetics.

(e) *True.* The proportionality is known as clearance and this remains constant under stable clinical conditions. The simple implication of this is that if the dose is doubled, the steady-state concentration is doubled, and if the dose is halved, the steady-state concentration is halved.

3 (a) *True.*   The proportion eliminated from the plasma is fixed, i.e. 50% will be removed per eight hours.

(b) *False.*   The proportion is constant or fixed, but the actual amount is not constant because, in first-order kinetics, the rate of elimination is proportional to the concentration. Thus, the initial high concentration will result in a greater amount being eliminated; in the first four hours about 29 mg will be eliminated.

(c) *True.*   The proportion is constant, half of the initial amount in the first eight hours (i.e. 50 mg) and half of the remainder in the next eight hours (i.e. 25 mg), totalling 75 mg.

(d) *False.*   The drug will not be absorbed instantaneously; time will elapse before the whole 100 mg enters the circulation. Additionally, absorption may well be less than 100%.

(e) *True.*   Twenty-four hours is three half-lives, i.e. $1/2 \times 1/2 \times 1/2 = 1/8$ will remain.

4 (a) *True.*   By definition.

(b) *False.*   A biexponential equation will often be necessary to characterize the processes of absorption and elimination (even in the absence of distribution effects) which are controlling the rise in plasma concentrations after oral administration. Therefore the defined kinetic model always describes the drug's elimination characteristics.

(c) *False.*⎫ If the rates of equilibration and the concentration gradi-
⎬ ents remain constant between plasma and tissues then a
(d) *False.*⎭ single-compartment model remains appropriate.

(e) *False.*   Highly protein-bound drugs are frequently characterized by single-compartment models, but this does not mean that all single-compartment drugs are highly protein-bound.

5 (a) *False.*   It is water-soluble, highly ionized drugs which do not readily penetrate the CNS.

(b) *True.*   For example, because of concentration in fat, propranolol has an apparent volume of distribution of 250 litres.

(c) *True.*   Lipid-soluble drugs are poorly ionized and therefore relatively readily cross cell membranes.

(d) *False.*   Following glomerular filtration, lipid-soluble drugs are readily reabsorbed by the renal tubule. Therefore they typically undergo hepatic metabolism to more water-soluble (ionized) molecules which can then be eliminated via the kidney.

(e) *False.*   Although lipid-soluble drugs are not readily eliminated unchanged via the kidney, they are often subject to extensive metabolism (by the liver).

6 (a) *False.* It is decreased in renal failure, mainly due to displacement by endogenous substances, but also to reduced plasma albumin concentration and altered affinity of the albumin molecule.

(b) *True.* Especially for acidic drugs.

(c) *True.* Lignocaine and other basic drugs bind to this acute-phase protein.

(d) *True.* This explains the potential for interactions involving displacement from binding sites.

(e) *False.* The opposite is true.

7 (a) *True.* ⎫ Enzyme activity is quantitatively increased (i.e. higher V_{max}) but there is no qualitative change (i.e. k_m un-

(b) *False.* ⎭ changed).

(c) *True.* Due to increased hepatic metabolism of the hormonal constituents.

(d) *False.*

(e) *True.* Autoinduction is an initial phenomenon during the first 1–2 weeks, and once a stable dose is established during long-term therapy there is no further need for a dosage increment.

8 (a) *True.* Alcohol is a mild inducer of hepatic enzyme activity.

(b) *False.* There is destruction of hepatocytes and vascular 'shunting', with reduction of total metabolizing capacity.

(c) *True.*

(d) *False.*

(e) *False.* It is only the use of antiepileptic therapy which causes induction of enzyme activity.

9 (a) *False.* The peak concentration is more directly related to the patient's volume of distribution, which may be dependent on age, sex, weight and height.

(b) *False.* The volume of distribution is a mathematical concept to denote the total volume of fluid throughout which the drug is distributed. Its calculation is based on the assumption that the concentration throughout is constant and is thus the same as is measured in the blood.

(c) *True.* These are the major organs of elimination.

(d) *True.*

(e) *True.* This is the concept of first-order kinetics. (NB Clearance is *constant* irrespective of the drug concentration.)

10 (a) *True.*   For example, phenytoin may be measured in the saliva.
     (b) *False.*   Oral absorption is usually good.
     (c) *True.*
     (d) *True.*   Lipid-soluble drugs typically are metabolized in the liver to water-soluble metabolites which are then eliminated via the kidney.
     (e) *False.*

Cardiovascular
Questions

11 **Antagonism (blockade) at beta-adrenoceptors:**
    (a)   Results in an increase in heart rate.
    (b)   Results in a decrease in blood pressure.
    (c)   Antagonizes some of the effects of noradrenaline and adrenaline.
— (d)   Causes vasodilatation of peripheral blood vessels.
    (e)   Is caused by prazosin.

12 **Beta-adrenoceptor antagonists are used in a variety of medical conditions:**
— (a)   In congestive cardiac failure (due to coronary artery disease) they usefully block the increased sympathetic drive.
    (b)   Their antihypertensive effect has a marked postural hypotensive component.
    (c)   In thyrotoxicosis, they can reduce muscle tremor.
— (d)   In the treatment of angina they dilate coronary arteries.
    (e)   They are useful as additional therapy for the relief of bronchospasm.

13 **The following mechanisms have been proposed as contributing to the antihypertensive effects of propranolol and atenolol:**
    (a)   Decreasing sympathetically mediated renin release.
    (b)   Increasing cardiac output.
    (c)   Effects on the central nervous system.
— (d)   Decreasing noradrenaline release from sympathetic nerve endings.
    (e)   Peripheral arteriolar vasodilatation.

14 **The following beta-blockers have these characteristics:**
    (a)   Propranolol does not cross the blood–brain barrier.
    (b)   Pindolol has significant partial agonist activity at beta-adrenoceptors.
    (c)   Metoprolol is cardioselective.
— (d)   Propranolol has powerful membrane stabilizing activity, which is the major component of its antiarrhythmic activity in clinical practice.
    (e)   Atenolol is eliminated primarily by the kidney.

15 Alpha-adrenoceptors:
(a) Are sub-classified in a similar way to beta-adrenoceptors i.e. alpha$_1$-receptors in the heart and alpha$_2$-receptors in other tissues, e.g. lung.
(b) The classical alpha-receptor is located post-junctionally on peripheral blood vessels and promotes vasoconstriction.
(c) Alpha-adrenoceptor antagonists have useful antihypertensive properties.
(d) Noradrenaline stimulates both alpha- and beta-adrenoceptors.
(e) Stimulation of alpha$_2$-adrenoceptors can reduce blood pressure.

16 Digoxin:
(a) Has positive inotropic activity.
(b) Inhibits central vagal connections and thus increases the heart rate.
(c) Inhibits Na^+/K^+ ATPase.
(d) Improves the blood supply to the myocardium.
(e) Has an atropine-like action on cholinergic receptors in the heart.

17 Toxicity with digoxin (and related cardiac glycosides):
(a) Is an infrequent complication, occurring in less than 1% of patients treated with the drug.
(b) Occurs more frequently in patients also treated with thiazide diuretics.
(c) Typically presents as a gastrointenstinal upset.
(d) Can cause a sudden fatal arrhythmia.
(e) Is more likely in patients with renal impairment.

18 The following are correct observations about the drugs used for the treatment of cardiac dysrhythmias:
(a) Quinidine and lignocaine share the property of membrane stabilizing activity.
(b) Drugs which exert membrane stabilizing activity prevent the conduction of propagated action potentials, but do not significantly affect resting membrane potential.
(c) Beta-adrenoceptor antagonists are particularly useful in treating the dysrhythmias associated with increased catecholamine activity.
(d) Amiodarone prolongs the action potential and increases the refractory period.
(e) The major action of verapamil is to slow conduction through the AV node.

19 In the treatment of cardiac dysrhythmias:
  (a) Lignocaine is best administered intravenously because it undergoes extensive first-pass hepatic metabolism following oral administration.
  (b) Phenytoin is useful in controlling dysrhythmias induced by digoxin toxicity.
  (c) Combined intravenous therapy with verapamil and a beta-blocker is safe and effective in all cases of paroxysmal atrial tachycardia.
  (d) Amiodarone has a wide range of antidysrhythmic activity and a very long plasma half-life.
  (e) A major part of the antidysrhythmic action of procainamide is due to its active metabolite, N-acetylprocainamide.

20 Lignocaine:
  (a) Is widely used as a local anaesthetic.
  (b) Does not penetrate the blood–brain barrier.
  (c) Reduces the maximum rate of depolarization of the myocardial cell membrane.
  (d) Has beta-adrenoceptor antagonist activity.
  (e) Has an antidysrhythmic mechanism of action similar to verapamil.

21 The antidysrhythmic drug, disopyramide:
  (a) May cause dry mouth and blurred vision.
  (b) Delays conduction along the bundle of His.
  (c) Is eliminated mainly by the kidney.
  (d) Is effective after both oral and intravenous administration.
  (e) Increases the force of cardiac contraction.

22 In normal therapeutic doses nifedipine, the calcium antagonist or slow calcium channel blocker:
  (a) Has a profound negative inotropic effect.
  (b) Should not be given with beta-blockers.
  (c) Is effective in the treatment of hypertension.
  (d) Frequently worsens intermittent claudication.
  (e) Has pronounced antiarrhythmic activity.

23 The following are correct observations about the use of vasodilator
    drugs in heart failure:
    (a) Arterial dilators act mainly on the skeletal muscle arteries.
    (b) Venodilators reduce venous return to the heart and thus reduce
         cardiac pre-load.
    (c) Nitrates act mainly on the arterial system.
    (d) Vasodilator therapy is not useful if the patient is already
         receiving digoxin.
    (e) ACE inhibitors have useful vasodilator effects on both arteries
         and veins.

24 In the treatment of severe acute heart failure:
    (a) Beta$_1$-adrenoceptor agonists promote myocardial inotropic
         activity.
    (b) Of the available beta$_1$ agonist drugs, dopamine is the most
         selective with no effects outside of the myocardium.
    (c) Bradydysrhythmias are recognized complications of treatment
         with dopamine.
    (d) Both dopamine and dobutamine are available for oral
         administration and have largely superseded digoxin in the
         chronic treatment of heart failure.
    (e) Beta$_1$-adrenoceptor agonist drugs are contraindicated in the
         setting of acute myocardial infarction.

25 In angina:
    (a) Glyceryl trinitrate is probably effective as a result of its
         peripheral vasodilator activity, resulting in reductions in cardiac
         pre-load and after-load.
    (b) Metoprolol is effective because it is an antagonist of peripheral
         beta$_2$-adrenoceptors and therefore reduces peripheral arterial
         resistance.
    (c) Dilatation of coronary arteries is the principal effect of long-
         term antianginal treatment with verapamil.
    (d) Isosorbide dinitrate is useful for long-term treatment because it
         has a relatively prolonged duration of action since it is
         eliminated mainly unchanged via the kidney.
    (e) Nifedipine is more effective than verapamil because it causes less
         reduction in the contractility of myocardial cells.

Cardiovascular
Answers

11 (a) *False.* It is a stimulation of beta-adrenoceptors which causes an increase in heart rate — directly via the cardiac $beta_1$-receptor and reflexly as a result of $beta_2$-mediated peripheral vasodilatation.

(b) *True.* The specific mechanisms underlying the anti-hypertensive effects remain unclear.

(c) *True.* Both these catecholamines have beta-adrenoceptor agonist activity.

(d) *False.* Although beta-blockers have an antihypertensive effect, antagonism of vascular $beta_2$-adrenoceptors facilitates peripheral vasoconstriction.

(e) *False.* Prazosin is an $alpha_1$-adrenoceptor antagonist.

12 (a) *False.* Blockade of sympathetic drive may precipitate or exacerbate cardiac failure.

(b) *False.* The necessary baroreceptor reflex-mediated vaso-constriction of resistance arterioles, which is dependent upon $alpha_1$-adrenoceptors, remains intact.

(c) *True.* Responsiveness to catecholamines is enhanced in thyrotoxicosis: skeletal muscle tremor is $beta_2$-adrenoceptor mediated.

(d) *False.* The antianginal effect is probably due to antagonism of the increase in heart rate and cardiac output which occurs in response to stress, exercise, anxiety, etc.

(e) *False.* The bronchial $beta_2$-adrenoceptor facilitates broncho-dilatation: $beta_2$-adrenoceptor antagonism may therefore precipitate bronchial constriction.

13 (a) *True.* Renin release is, in part, beta-adrenoceptor mediated. It remains controversial whether the receptor is $beta_1$ or $beta_2$ subtype.

(b) *False.* Increased cardiac output results from beta-adrenoceptor stimulation.

(c) *True.* By reducing sympathetic outflow from the CNS.

(d) *True.* The control of noradrenaline release from sympathetic neurones is modulated by presynaptic $alpha_2$-adrenoceptors (decrease) and $beta_2$-adrenoceptors (increase).

(e) *False.*

Propanolol

14 (a) *False.* It is highly lipophilic and so it readily penetrates the CNS. This may contribute to both its effects (central reduction of sympathetic tone) and side-effects (vivid dreams). Atenolol is least lipophilic.

(b) *True.* This effect, which is also referred to as intrinsic sympathomimetic activity (ISA), is also seen with oxprenolol.

(c) *True.* Metoprolol and atenolol are both cardioselective, i.e. $beta_1$ selective. (NB Cardioselectivity is not absolute.)

(d) *False.* Significant degrees of membrane stabilizing or quinidine-like or local anaesthetic activity are seen only at toxic doses.

(e) *True* In contrast to propranolol and metoprolol, for example, which undergo extensive first-pass hepatic metabolism.

15 (a) *False.* This classification distinguishes the subtypes of beta-adrenoceptors but alpha-adrenoceptors are not classed according to tissues or organs.

(b) *True.* This is the basis of the classification for alpha-adrenoceptors. $Alpha_2$-adrenoceptors are located at other sites in the nervous system, e.g. prejunctionally on sympathetic nerves.

(c) *True.* Prazosin is the best-known antihypertensive drug which acts as a selective antagonist at peripheral $alpha_1$-adrenoceptors.

(d) *True.* Although its alpha-adrenoceptor agonist activity is relatively more potent.

(e) *True.* Stimulation of the (inhibitory) $alpha_2$-adrenoceptors in the CNS/brain stem reduces sympathetic tone. *eg. clonidine, methyl dopa.*

16 (a) *True.* It has a positive inotropic action, because it increases the availability of intracellular calcium for the contractile mechanism.

(b) *False.* It promotes vagal activity both directly and centrally via an action in the medulla, and so tends to reduce heart rate.

(c) *True.* Membrane ATPase is responsible for the expulsion of intracellular Na^+ in exchange for K^+. Normally intracellular accumulation of Na^+ (and depletion of K^+) facilitates Ca^{2+} mobilization and the contractile processes.

(d) *False.* Digoxin has no direct effect on coronary arteries.

(e) *False.* Digoxin slows heart rate via mechanisms of vagal stimulation. This would be antagonized by atropine.

17 (a) *False.* Digoxin has a low therapeutic ratio and toxicity is a relatively frequent complication.

(b) *True.* Digoxin's effects on Na^+/K^+ ATPase cause intracellular K^+ depletion which leads to increased excitability of cardiac muscle. The hypokalaemia associated with diuretics potentiates this effect.

(c) *True.* Typically anorexia, nausea and vomiting.

(d) *True.* Increased ventricular excitability and automaticity may give rise to paroxysmal ventricular tachycardia and may lead to ventricular fibrillation.

(e) *True.* Elimination of digoxin is primarily dependent upon glomerular filtration: in moderate to severe degrees of renal failure the plasma half-life may increase 2–5-fold.

18 (a) *True.* According to the Vaughan Williams classification, drugs with membrane stabilizing activity constitute class I. These drugs also have local anaesthetic activity.

(b) *True.* Class I drugs all demonstrate these effects. The class may be further subdivided according to their effects on the duration of the action potential.

(i) Quinidine, disopyramide, procainamide are class Ia:
lengthen the action potential.
(ii) Lignocaine, tocainide, mexililine, phenytoin are class Ib:
shorten the action potential.
(iii) Flecainide, encainide, lorcainide are class Ic:
no effect on the action potential.

(c) *True.* The beta-blocker group form class II. They have weak membrane stabilizing activity which is not significant in usual therapeutic doses.

(d) *True.* This drug forms class III.

(e) *True.* This is the most important antidysrhythmic property of verapamil which is in class IV. It additionally inhibits calcium transport across the myocardial cell membrane.

19 (a) *True.* Lignocaine is 90–100% metabolized in the liver following oral administration. The lignocaine analogue, tocainide, may be used as oral therapy because it does not undergo first-pass metabolism.

(b) *True.*

(c) *False.* Severe hypotension and profound depression of atrioventricular conduction, leading to asystole, is a significant risk of this combination which is thus contraindicated.

(d) *True.* Its plasma half-life is greater than four weeks: it is usually reserved for dysrhythmias which have proved refractory to other treatments.

(e) *True.*

20 (a) *True.* It is widely used for this purpose, in concentrations about 10-fold greater than are used for antidysrhythmic effects. It blocks nerve impulses by preventing depolarization.

(b) *False.* It readily enters the CNS: mental confusion, hallucinations and convulsions are recognized toxic effects.

(c) *True.* It interferes with the maximum rate of depolarization and also with the threshold potential.

(d) *False.* It has no adrenergic actions: it affects cardiac electrical activity.

(e) *False.* Verapamil inhibits myocardial calcium entry (class IV antiarrhythmic). Lignocaine is a class I, i.e. membrane stabilizing.

21 (a) *True.* It has anticholinergic properties: thus, it also causes urinary retention.

(b) *True.* This is a feature of membrane-stabilizing drugs (class I).

(c) *True.* Dosage adjustment may be required if there is renal impairment.

(d) *True.*

(e) *False.* All drugs of this type depress cardiac contractility to some extent. Disopyramide has a well-recognized negative inotropic effect, even at low doses.

22 (a) *False.* This effect is obtained with nifedipine *in vitro* but only at very high concentrations which are not achieved *in vivo*.

(b) *False.* It may usefully be combined with beta-blockers both in hypertension and in angina.

(c) *True.*

(d) *False.* It may have a beneficial effect in the treatment of peripheral vascular disorders.

(e) *False.* This property is not a feature of nifedipine or other dihydropyridines, but is seen with verapamil.

23 (a) *False.* Arterial dilatation affects mainly the resistance vessels and the splanchnic circulation.

(b) *True.* ⎱ Nitrates act mainly on the venous system to reduce
(c) *False.* ⎰ cardiac pre-load.

(d) *False.* There is no contraindication to combined treatment with digoxin and a vasodilator. In many instances the combination is advantageous.

(e) *True.* ACE inhibitors (captopril and enalapril) have predominantly arteriolar effects, but they do also act on venous tone. They are particularly useful when the renin–angiotensin–aldosterone axis is stimulated.

24 (a) *True.* The drugs most frequently used in this context are dopamine and dobutamine.

(b) *False.* Dobutamine is a more selective beta$_1$ agonist than dopamine, which stimulates dopamine receptors in the kidney to increase renal blood flow (at low dose rates) and also acts on alpha-adrenoceptors to cause vasoconstriction and a slight rise in blood pressure (at high dose rates).

(c) *False.* Excessive stimulation of beta$_1$-receptors results in tachydysrhythmias.

(d) *False.* One of the disadvantages of beta-adrenoceptor agonists in heart failure is the lack of a suitable orally effective preparation.

(e) *False.*

25 (a) *True.* Generally the nitrates are effective in angina as a result of their venodilator action, which reduces cardiac pre-load: in special circumstances, either direct administration into the coronary arteries or during the course of high-dose intravenous therapy, there may be a direct coronary arterial vasodilator effect.

(b) *False.* Metoprolol is a selective $beta_1$-adrenoceptor antagonist. Blockade of $beta_2$-adrenoceptors in the peripheral blood vessels is of course associated with an increase in peripheral arterial resistance.

(c) *True.* Decreased tone in vascular smooth muscle cells, including coronary arteries, is the basis for the antianginal effects of calcium antagonists.

(d) *False.* Isosorbide dinitrate is extensively metabolized both in the liver and in the plasma itself.

(e) *False.*

Haematology
Questions

26 Blood clotting:
(a) In vitro is prevented by coumarin anticoagulants.
(b) Is impaired in severe vitamin K deficiency.
(c) Is prevented both in vivo and in vitro by heparin.
(d) Is prevented by heparin principally by inhibition of thrombin activation.
(e) Is impaired by aspirin.

27 The oral anticoagulant, warfarin:
(a) Is effective within about two hours of oral administration.
(b) Can be displaced from plasma protein binding sites by aspirin.
(c) Has useful in vitro activity.
(d) Has fibrinolytic activity.
(e) Will show a reduced anticoagulant effect if the patient begins treatment with a drug with hepatic enzyme-inducing activity.

28 Heparin is an anticoagulant which:
(a) Is destroyed in the gastrointestinal tract.
(b) Produces its anticoagulant effect primarily by reducing platelet adhesiveness.
(c) Is found naturally in mast cells.
(d) Has its action antagonized by protamine.
(e) Has its action antagonized by vitamin K.

29 In the treatment of iron deficiency anaemia:
(a) Intravenous iron therapy should be given to produce a rapid rise in haemoglobin in severe anaemia.
(b) Oral iron therapy produces an increase in haemoglobin of approximately 1 g/dl per week.
(c) Ferrous salts are more readily absorbed than ferric salts.
(d) Oral administration of ferrous salts frequently causes gastro-intestinal side-effects.
(e) Treatment has to be given for life.

30 The following observations about haematinic therapy are correct:

(a) Folic acid is absorbed only from the distal segment of the terminal ileum.

(b) To facilitate absorption from the injection site vitamin B_{12} must be administered as a combined preparation with intrinsic factor.

(c) Both folic acid and iron supplements may temporarily be required during pregnancy.

(d) In the treatment of pernicious anaemia, vitamin B_{12} injections require to be continued lifelong.

(e) Co-trimoxazole is contraindicted in patients receiving folic acid supplements because it interferes with folate utilization.

Haematology
Answers

26 (a) *False.* These drugs only work in *vivo*: their action depends on inhibiting the synthesis of clotting factors in the liver.

(b) *True.* Vitamin K is a necessary co-factor for the hepatic synthesis of clotting factors.

(c) *True.* Heparin inhibits a number of coagulation steps, particularly activation of thrombin, and therefore is effective both in *vivo* and in *vitro*.

(d) *True.*

(e) *True.* Low-dosage aspirin (<150 mg daily) inhibits platelet aggregation by selectively interfering with platelet cyclo-oxygenase.

27 (a) *False.* It acts as a competitive inhibitor opposing the hepatic synthesis of the vitamin K-dependent clotting factors. It typically takes about 48 hours before a reduction in the levels of clotting factors is apparent in the blood.

(b) *True.* The displacement leads to an increased availability of 'free' warfarin and to an increased anticoagulant effect.

(c) *False.* Its action depends on interfering with the hepatic synthesis of the vitamin K-dependent clotting factors II (prothrombin), VII, IX, and X.

(d) *False.*

(e) *True.* Induction of hepatic enzyme activity (e.g. by phenytoin or phenobarbitone) results in a more rapid metabolism (elimination) of warfarin with a consequent reduction in its effect.

28 (a) *True.* Obviously, therefore, requires to be administered parenterally.

(b) *False.* The strongly electronegative heparin radicles inhibit many sequences in the clotting mechanism, in particular thromboplastin and thrombin generation. In low doses, heparin has a weak antiplatelet aggregation effect.

(c) *True.* It is a naturally occurring mucopolysaccharide found in mast cells, particularly in the lung. Its physiological function is unknown.

(d) *True.* Approximately 1 mg intravenous protamine, which is a protein with a strong positive charge, will immediately neutralize 100 units of heparin.

(e) *False.* It is the anticoagulant effect of warfarin which is antagonized by vitamin K. This is not an immediate effect.

29 (a) *False.* The limiting factor is the rate of synthesis of haemoglobin by bone marrow. For this purpose iron is equally readily available following oral therapy.

(b) *True.* This means that the haemoglobin level is usually satisfactorily restored within 1–2 months. To replenish iron stores in addition a total of six months' iron therapy is recommended.

(c) *True.* The absorption of *ferrous* ions involves uptake by the carrier protein transferrin, whereas *ferric* ions are bound to ferritin within the columnar cells which are duly lost in faeces.

(d) *True.* The side-effects of nausea and epigastric discomfort and upset bowel habit occur in about 20% of patients and seem to be related to the total available amounts of iron.

(e) *False.* See (b).

30 (a) *False.* Folic acid is absorbed from the upper small intestine. It is the absorption of vitamin B_{12} which is confined to the terminal ileum.

(b) *False.* The lack of intrinsic factor prevents absorption from the gastrointestinal tract.

(c) *True.* Due to the requirements of the fetus and the lack of long-term body stores.

(d) *True.*

(e) *False.* Co-trimoxazole inhibits folate synthesis in bacteria: this is not relevant for folate administration.

Respiratory
Questions

31 The beta-adrenoceptor agonist, salbutamol:
   (a) Has no effect on the heart rate, even at high dose.
   (b) Causes contraction of uterine smooth muscle.
   (c) Causes bronchodilatation.
   (d) Can provoke skeletal muscle tremor.
   (e) Selectively and specifically stimulates beta$_2$-adrenoceptors in the airways.

32 Aminophylline:
   (a) Can stimulate the CNS.
   (b) Can increase intracellular levels of cyclic AMP.
   (c) Can competitively antagonize the effects of ADP.
   (d) Has a bronchodilator effect.
   (e) Is free of cardiac effects.

33 The following drugs have a role in relieving bronchospasm:
   (a) Beta$_2$-adrenoceptor agonists.
   (b) Histamine H$_1$-receptor blockers.
   (c) Inhibitors of prostaglandin synthesis.
   (d) Calcium channel blockers.
   (e) Anticholinergic (muscarinic) drugs.

34 Sodium cromoglycate:
   (a) Is well absorbed from the gastrointestinal tract.
   (b) Stabilizes mast cells and prevents their degranulation.
   (c) Is particularly useful in childhood asthma.
   (d) Is most useful for the relief of acute bronchospasm.
   (e) Is useful in the treatment of allergic rhinitis.

35 The following considerations apply to the administration of aminophylline:
   (a) A rapid (30 seconds) bolus intravenous injection is the optimum mode of administration.
   (b) It is contraindicated in patients already receiving salbutamol.
   (c) The dose is likely to require reduction if the patient is known to have hepatic impairment.
   (d) The dose should be increased if the patient has been receiving maintenance theophylline therapy.
   (e) Oral and intravenous administration are equally effective.

36 In the treatment of status asthmaticus:
  (a) High-concentration oxygen therapy is indicated.
  (b) Salbutamol is best administered as an aerosol from a nebulizer in the oxygen flow.
  —(c) The effects of intravenous hydrocortisone in relieving bronchospasm will be apparent within 30 minutes of administration.
  (d) Opiate analgesics should be used routinely to relieve distress.
  —(e) Artificial ventilation is contraindicated.

37 Therapy with a high concentration of oxygen:
  (a) Is likely to cause carbon dioxide narcosis in a previously fit young man with post-operative pneumonia.
  (b) Is contraindicated in acute pulmonary oedema.
  (c) Is necessary for patients with a low arterial Pco_2.
  (d) Is provided by a 24% or 28% controlled oxygen mask.
  (e) Is contraindicated in acute exacerbations of chronic bronchitis.

38 Naloxone:
  (a) Is a relatively pure agonist at opiate receptors.
  (b) Has pronounced analgesic activity.
  (c) May facilitate the withdrawal of morphine or heroin in addicts.
  (d) Is effective in reversing the respiratory depressant effect of alcohol.
  (e) Is less effective as a respiratory stimulant than nalorphine.

39 In the treatment of pulmonary tuberculosis:
  (a) Isoniazid and rifampicin are bactericidal.
  (b) Peripheral neuropathy may complicate the use of isoniazid: this can be prevented by pyridoxine.
  (c) Ototoxicity is a well-recognized adverse effect of rifampicin.
  (d) Combination regimens are indicated to limit the development of bacterial resistance.
  (e) The preferred current practice is for a triple-drug regimen to be maintained for not less than two years.

40 Stimulation of the respiratory centre in the CNS occurs with:
  (a) Nikethamide.
  (b) Alcohol.
  (c) Carbon dioxide.
  (d) Doxapram.
  (e) Diazepam.

Respiratory
Answers

31 (a) *False.* Salbutamol selectively activates beta$_2$-adrenoceptors, but the selectivity is not absolute and at high doses cardiac beta$_1$-receptors will also be activated.

(b) *False.* Activation of beta$_2$-adrenoceptors relaxes uterine smooth muscle: thus, beta$_2$ agonist drugs may be used to control premature labour.

(c) *True.* Bronchodilation is salbutamol's major therapeutic use but the oral doses necessary to produce this effect invariably cause systemic effects, including cardio-

(d) *True.* stimulation (beta$_1$) and muscle tremor (beta$_2$).

(e) *False.* Inhalation is thus the preferred route of administration.

32 (a) *True.* This is a general property of the methylxanthine group which also includes theophylline and caffeine.

(b) *True.* Due to inhibition of the enzyme phosphodiesterase which inactivates cyclic AMP. However, this effect is seen with concentrations higher than are usually obtained *in vivo*.

(c) *True.* The adenosine compounds are mediators of response (in this case, constriction of bronchial smooth muscle) and their effects are competitively antagonized by methylxanthines.

(d) *True.*

(e) *False.* Tachycardia and ventricular dysrhythmias may occur. Attributed to a 'direct' effect on the heart, perhaps interference with intracellular calcium handling.

33 (a) *True.* As above for salbutamol: fenoterol and terbutaline are other beta$_2$ agonists.

(b) *False.* Although histamine, prostaglandins and other bronchoconstrictor substances are involved in allergic asthma,

(c) *False.* these individual treatments are ineffective.

(d) *True.* Blockade of alpha-mediated bronchoconstrictor influences will facilitate beta$_2$-mediated bronchodilatation, but systemic side-effects override the respiratory effects.

(e) *True.* However, given systemically the side-effects are troublesome: ipratropium by inhalation is particularly useful in older patients with obstructive airways disease.

34 (a) *False.* It is destroyed in the stomach: requires to be administered by inhalation.

   (b) *True.* Therefore the release of histamine and other bronchoconstrictor substances is prevented. It is therefore best used prophylactically.

   (c) *True.* The allergic component is more pronounced.

   (d) *False.* Its role is to prevent histamine release. Once bronchospasm is established it is ineffective.

   (e) *True.* As prophylaxis.

35 (a) *False.* Rapid intravenous administration of the drug can produce a direct cardiotoxic effect with tachycardia or ventricular ectopic activity.

   (b) *False.*

   (c) *True.*

   (d) *False.* Toxicity, particularly CNS effects, is associated with high blood levels.

   (e) *False.* Aminophylline itself is intensely irritant to the gastric mucosa.

36 (a) *True.* Chronic CO_2 retention is not a feature of asthma. Acute CO_2 narcosis may occur in life-threateningly severe acute asthmatic attacks when acute respiratory failure supervenes.

   (b) *True.* The patient is usually unable to control and time his respiration to allow appropriate use of the standard inhaler.

   (c) *False.* The effects of corticosteroids are delayed in onset, typically by 4–6 hours.

   (d) *False.* Although respiratory depression is not typical of asthma there is sufficient danger from the use of opiates that they should be avoided.

   (e) *False.* In very severe status asthmaticus artificial ventilation may be necessary to sustain life.

37 (a) *False.*

   (b) *False.*

   (c) *False.*

   (d) *False.*

   (e) *True.* The chronic CO_2 retention leads to the respiratory drive being dependent upon hypoxia. Accordingly high-concentration therapy will improve the hypoxia with the risk of depressing the respiratory drive.

38 (a) *True.*   Naloxone is classified as a specific opioid antagonist
                     without agonist activity.

   (b) *False.*   It has no significant analgesic activity.

   (c) *False.*   If administered to an opiate addict it may precipitate an
                     acute withdrawal syndrome.

   (d) *False.*

   (e) *False.*   Naloxone is not a direct respiratory stimulant but it
                     contrasts with nalorphine which is not a pure opiate
                     antagonist but which has some agonist activity and may
                     therefore cause respiratory depression.

39 (a) *True.*   Of the first-line antituberculous drugs isoniazid,
                     rifampicin and pyrazinamide are bactericidal, whereas
                     ethambutol is bacteriostatic.

   (b) *True.*   The side-effect of peripheral neuropathy is most likely to
                     occur in slow acetylators and can be prevented by the
                     prophylactic co-administration of pyridoxine.

   (c) *False.*   Ototoxicity is the main adverse reaction attributable to
                     streptomycin. The major adverse effect of rifampicin is
                     hepatitis.

   (d) *True.* ⎫ Typical combination regimen with isoniazid, rifampicin
                     and either ethambutol or pyrazinamide is administered
                     initially for eight weeks for the treatment of pulmonary
                     tuberculosis. Subsequently for up to six months isoni-
   (e) *False.* ⎭ azid and rifampicin are given.

40 (a) *True.*   This is a general CNS stimulant and is virtually obsolete
                     because of the risk of provoking convulsions.

   (b) *False.*

   (c) *True.*   Physiologically the partial pressure of CO_2 controls the
                     respiratory drive.

   (d) *True.*   This is analeptic therapy, similar to nikethamide but
                     with slightly reduced risk of provoking convulsions.

   (e) *False.*

Gastrointestinal
Questions

41 The following statements about antacids are correct:
    (a) Aluminium hydroxide enhances the absorption of oxytetracycline.
    (b) The excessive consumption of sodium bicarbonate can cause systemic alkalosis.
    (c) Symptomatic improvement is achieved only when large acid-neutralizing doses are administered.
    (d) Magnesium trisilicate can cause constipation.
    (e) Although they provide symptomatic relief, they are of no value in the healing of duodenal ulcers.

42 Cimetidine:
    (a) Reduces gastric acid secretion induced by pentagastrin.
    (b) Has anticholinergic activity.
    (c) Blocks histamine H_2-receptors.
    (d) Raises the pH of gastric acid secretion.
    (e) Reduces the volume of gastric acid secretion.

43 The treatment of gastric ulcers with carbenoxolone:
    (a) Reduces the volume and hydrogen ion content of gastric acid secretion.
    (b) Is compromised if spironolactone is administered concurrently.
    (c) Increases the rate of gastric emptying.
    (d) Increases mucus production in the stomach.
    (e) Can cause side-effects due to sodium and fluid retention.

44 Treatment of peptic ulcers with:
    (a) Propantheline produces H_2-receptor blockade.
    (b) Cimetidine inhibits pentagastrin-induced gastric acid secretion.
    (c) Ranitidine is associated with antiandrogenic effects.
    (d) Sucralfate is associated with powerful antacid activity.
    (e) Carbenoxolone is associated with suppression of acid secretion.

45 In the management of gastric ulcers:
    (a) Cimetidine is more effective than bed rest.
    (b) Aspirin is a good analgesic.
    (c) Corticosteroids are beneficial.
    (d) Carbenoxolone is perfectly safe.
    (e) Tobacco smoking delays healing.

46 The following drugs are particularly useful in the treatment of motion sickness:
   (a) Hyoscine.
   (b) Ranitidine.
   (c) Promethazine.
   (d) Levodopa.
   (e) Metoclopramide.

47 Metoclopramide:
   (a) Is well-recognized as causing Parkinsonian-like symptoms, particularly in children.
   (b) Is used to treat duodenal ulcers.
   (c) Promotes gastric emptying.
   (d) Is useful in treating vomiting following cancer chemotherapy.
   (e) Acts directly on the gastric mucosa.

48 The following adverse effects on the GI system are well recognized to be due to the associated drug:
   (a) Pseudomembranous colitis with clindamycin.
   (b) Diarrhoea with ampicillin.
   (c) Hepatotoxicity with isoniazid.
   (d) Cirrhosis with methotrexate.
   (e) Constipation with atenolol.

49 Sulphasalazine is used in the treatment of ulcerative colitis:
   (a) Sulphasalazine is a combination of sulphapyridine and 5-aminosalicylic acid.
   (b) 5-Aminosalicylic acid is thought to be the active component by virtue of its local anti-inflammatory effects on the colonic mucosa.
   (c) Sulphapyridine is absorbed from the GI tract and is metabolized in the liver.
   (d) Side-effects of nausea and vomiting are well recognized.
   (e) The use of sulphasalazine is contraindicated if corticosteroids are also being administered.

50 The following observations about altered bowel habits are correct:
   (a) Codeine phosphate is useful treatment for the diarrhoea associated with diverticular disease.
   (b) Mebeverine is an antispasmodic agent employed in the treatment of the irritable bowel syndrome.
   (c) The long-term use of liquid paraffin is associated with malabsorption of fat-soluble vitamins.
   (d) Diphenoxylate is an opiate derivative which reduces intestinal motility.
   (e) Loperamide has anticholinergic activity and is therefore a useful antidiarrhoeal drug.

Gastrointestinal
Answers

41 (a) *False.* Chelates are formed between tetracylines and Al^{3+} salts (also Ca^{2+}, Mg^{2+}) and absorption is reduced.

(b) *True.* It is soluble and is absorbed into the systemic circulation.

(c) *False.* Symptomatic improvement occurs even with small doses.

(d) *False.* Salts of Mg^{2+} act as an osmotic purgative and so cause diarrhoea. Salts of Al^{3+} tend to constipate.

(e) *False.* In placebo-controlled studies there is an increased rate of ulcer healing.

42 (a) *True.* The histamine (H_2) receptor is thought to mediate a final common pathway for acid secretion following a variety of stimuli.

(b) *False.* Although it does reduce the acid secretion arising from cholinergic stimulation.

(c) *True.* It is a selective H_2-receptor antagonist.

(d) *True.* By inhibiting physiological secretion of gastric acid.

(e) *True.*

43 (a) *False.* Its action depends on promoting gastric mucosal resistance.

(b) *True.* Spironolactone and amiloride both interfere with its ulcer-healing effect.

(c) *False.* It has no direct effect on gastric motility.

(d) *True.* This is a component of its mucosal protective effect.

(e) *True.* It has a steroid structure similar to aldosterone and so causes Na^+ retention and K^+ loss via the kidney.

44 (a) *False.* This is an anticholinergic drug.

(b) *True.* Both basal and stimulated acid production is reduced.

(c) *False.* Antiandrogenic effects, particularly gynaecomastia, are recognized to occur with cimetidine but not with ranitidine.

(d) *False.* It has minimal antacid properties and seems to act as a gastric mucosal protective.

(e) *False.* It has no effect on gastric acid output, and probably acts to protect the mucosa.

31

45 (a) *True.*

(b) *False.* The local effects of salicylates on gastric mucosa interfere with ulcer healing and may precipitate bleeding.

(c) *False.* They interfere with healing and may precipitate bleeding.

(d) *True.* Because of a 'protective' effect on the gastric mucosa.

(e) *True.* Both bed rest and cessation of smoking are useful adjunctive therapies for resistant cases.

46 (a) *True.* It is an anticholinergic drug and it acts by a central action on the vomiting centre in the medulla.

(b) *False.* It is an H_2-receptor antagonist.

(c) *True.* Because of its anticholinergic properties.

(d) *False.* It is used in the treatment of Parkinsonism: anorexia and vomiting are recognized side-effects.

(e) *False.* Although it is a useful antiemetic its central action is primarily on the chemoreceptor trigger zone; thus it is more effective against drug or metabolic causes of vomiting.

47 (a) *True.* Related to a dopamine antagonist effect in the CNS.

(b) *False.* It has no effect on ulcer healing, or acid production.

(c) *True.* This contributes to its antiemetic effect.

(d) *True.* In this circumstance it has been successfully used in very high doses.

(e) *False.* A central dopamine receptor antagonist acting at chemoreceptor trigger zone.

48 (a) *True.* Diarrhoea is a relatively common side-effect of broad-spectrum antimicrobials, particularly ampicillin and its derivatives, and is usually attributed to overgrowth of gut organisms. The more serious and potentially fatal complication of pseudomembranous colitis (due to a toxin released by *Clostridium difficile*) occurs rarely with antimicrobials, including ampicillin, but is a particular feature of lincomycin and clindamycin whose

(b) *True.* use has therefore been restricted.

(c) *True.* Minor abnormalities in up to 20% of patients but hepatic necrosis in only 0·1%. Probably related to the production of a reactive intermediate metabolite and occurs more commonly in fast acetylators and with concomitant enzyme-inducing drugs, especially rifampicin.

(d) *True.* Especially of underlying hepatic disease: dose-related.

(e) *False.*

49 (a) *True.*

(b) *True.* The 5-aminosalicylic acid is only poorly absorbed from the GI tract.

(c) *True.* Sulphapyridine is absorbed from the GI tract and metabolized in the liver. Accumulation of sulpha-pyridine is more likely to occur in slow acetylators and gives rise to side-effects of nausea and vomiting. In males reversible infertility is also a well-recognized side-effect.

(d) *True.*

(e) *False.* The anti-inflammatory activities of the two drugs are via different mechanisms and they can therefore be used in combination.

50 (a) *False.* Codeine raises intracolonic pressure and increases sphincter tone and so it should be avoided in diverticular disease.

(b) *True.* The pathophysiology of the irritable bowel syndrome is poorly understood but episodes of intestinal spasm are thought to contribute. Mebeverine is an antispasmodic agent.

(c) *True.*

(d) *True.* By its action on the myenteric plexus.

(e) *True.*

Endocrine
Questions

51 **The following are recognized complications of hormonal oral contraceptives:**
(a) Osteomalacia.
(b) Peripheral neuropathy.
(c) Hemiplegia.
(d) Inappropriate ADH secretion.
(e) Hypertension.

52 **In combined hormonal oral contraceptives, oestrogens:**
(a) Inhibit release of luteinizing hormone (LH).
(b) Inhibit release of follicle stimulating hormone (FSH).
(c) Cause increased risk of blood clotting.
(d) Cause thickening of cervical mucus.
(e) Are associated with ovarian carcinoma.

53 **Corticosteroids with glucocorticoid activity:**
(a) Include beclomethasone.
(b) Have an almost immediate bronchodilator effect in the treatment of status asthmaticus.
(c) Do not have anti-inflammatory activity.
(d) Are devoid of mineralocorticoid activity.
(e) When given by inhalation do not significantly affect pituitary function.

54 **Hydrocortisone:**
(a) Is formed in the liver from cortisone which is synthesized in the adrenal cortex.
(b) Has purely mineralocorticoid activity.
(c) Does not suppress the hypothalamic–pituitary–adrenal axis.
(d) Has no actions in the CNS.
(e) Very rarely causes side-effects in the long term.

55 **Aldosterone:**
(a) Action on the kidney is blocked competitively by triamterene.
(b) Secretion is indirectly controlled by renin release from the kidney.
(c) Secretion leads to K^+ retention by the renal tubules.
(d) Secretion is increased by infusions of isotonic sodium chloride.
(e) Is synthesized in the adrenal gland.

56 Significant interactions with the combined oral contraceptives have been demonstrated with:
   (a) Warfarin.
   (b) Rifampicin.
   (c) Aspirin.
   (d) Diazepam.
   (e) Phenytoin.

57 Insulin:
   (a) Is synthesized in the beta-cells of the islets of Langerhans in the pancreas.
   (b) Is effective orally when combined with zinc.
   (c) Promotes the uptake of glucose into cells.
   (d) Has its actions opposed by glucagon.
   (e) Has its actions potentiated by non-selective beta-adrenoceptor blockers.

58 Carbimazole diminishes thyroid function by:
   (a) Preventing tri-iodothyronine (T_3) and thyroxine (T_4) release.
   (b) Inhibiting formation of iodinated residues.
   (c) Preventing iodine uptake by the gland.
   (d) Producing thyroid atrophy.
   (e) Inhibiting organic combination of iodine.

59 Oral hypoglycaemic (antidiabetic) drugs:
   (a) Fall into two main categories: sulphonylureas and biguanides.
   (b) Are best used as an alternative to dietary carbohydrate restriction.
   (c) Cannot produce symptomatic hypoglycaemia.
   (d) Act mainly by augmenting the actions of insulin.
   (e) May be used for mild cases of diabetic ketoacidosis.

60 Chlorpropamide:
   (a) Is a long-acting sulphonylurea.
   (b) Is metabolized and inactivated by the liver.
   (c) Is particularly useful in the elderly.
   (d) Interacts with alcohol to cause profound facial flushing.
   (e) Is associated with the serious side-effect of lacticacidosis.

Endocrine
Answers

51 (a) *False.*
  (b) *False.*
  (c) *True.* Associated with the thrombotic effects of oestrogen.
  (d) *False.*
  (e) *True.* Probably related to sodium retention and altered vascular reactivity.

52 (a) *False.* The progestogen component inhibits LH release.
  (b) *True.* The administration of exogenous oestrogens by means of the natural feedback mechanisms inhibits the release of both LH and FSH.
  (c) *True.* This seems to be particularly associated with the oestrogen component.
  (d) *False.* This is an effect of progestogens, and is probably the major mechanism of the progestogen-only pill.
  (e) *False.* Use of the combined pill seems to protect against ovarian carcinoma.

53 (a) *True.* It is a powerful anti-inflammatory synthetic steroid usually administered by metered aerosol inhaler to reduce the risk of systemic side-effects.
  (b) *False.* Their effects are complex, but include reduction of the release of bronchoconstrictor substances. This is ineffective against established bronchospasm, but they appear to enhance the responsiveness to other bronchodilator drugs, particularly $beta_2$ agonists.
  (c) *False.* Anti-inflammatory activity and glucocorticoid activity are inseparable.
  (d) *False.* The synthetic glucocorticoids are virtually free of mineralocorticoid activity but prednisolone and hydrocortisone have significant mineralocorticoid effects.
  (e) *True.* A small amount of inhaled steroid is available systematically but is usually insufficient to suppress ACTH secretion.

54 (a) *True.*

(b) *False.* It has a ratio of glucocorticoid to mineralocorticoid of 25:1.

(c) *False.* All systemic glucocorticosteriods do.

(d) *False.* Euphoria is a well-recognized 'benefit' and overt psychoses occur.

(e) *False.* The use of even 'physiological' doses is associated with side-effects in the long term.

55 (a) *False.* Spironolactone is the potassium-sparing diuretic drug which acts as a competitive antagonist of aldosterone.

(b) *True.* Increased renin activity promotes the production of angiotensin II which stimulates aldosterone release from the adrenal gland.

(c) *False.* Aldosterone's effects are Na^+ (and water) retention and K^+ loss.

(d) *False.* Excess sodium or increased circulating fluid volume depresses renin activity and thereby decreases aldosterone release.

(e) *True.*

56 (a) *False.*

(b) *True.* Rifampicin induces hepatic enzyme activity, leading to more rapid metabolism of the hormones, with consequent lessening of efficacy.

(c) *False.*

(d) *False.*

(e) *True.* It is also an enzyme inducer.

57 (a) *True.*

(b) *False.* It is a peptide and, whether or not it is combined with zinc, it is degraded in the upper GI tract.

(c) *True.* To form glycogen (in muscle) and fat (in adipose tissue).

(d) *True.* Glucagon acts to increase blood glucose, mainly by glycogenolysis in the liver.

(e) *True.* The hypoglycaemic response to insulin causes $beta_2$-mediated glycogenolysis in the liver.

58 (a) *False.* Carbimazole has no effect on the release/secretion of thyroid hormone and so it takes approximately three weeks until its effect is apparent and hormone stores have been depleted.

    (b) *True.*

    (c) *False.* Interference with the uptake of iodine into the thyroid gland is a feature of potassium perchlorate which is now rarely used.

    (d) *False.*

    (e) *True.* Carbimazole (and its active metabolite methimazole) and propylthiouracil affect thyroid hormone synthesis by interfering with the formation of iodinated tyrosine residues and with the coupling/combination of the iodotyrosines.

59 (a) *True.* Sulphonylureas (e.g. chlorpropamide, glibenclamide) form the main group: the only biguanide is metformin.

    (b) *False.* Diet is crucial in the management of the maturity-onset type of diabetes: oral hypoglycaemic drugs should be used to augment dietary restriction.

    (c) *False.* This may occur if a meal is missed or if the dose is excessive, and especially with the long-acting types, particularly chlorpropamide.

    (d) *True.* Sulphonylureas were originally thought to stimulate insulin production/release from the pancreas but they also act to 'sensitize' insulin receptors in various organs and tissues. The biguanide metformin acts to increase peripheral glucose utilization and decrease glucose absorption from the GI tract.

    (e) *False.* They are contraindicated (and ineffective) in this circumstance: insulin is required.

60 (a) *True.* It is eliminated mainly by the kidney and has a half-life of more than 24 hours. It is suitable for once-daily administration.

    (b) *False.* It is renally eliminated. Most other sulphonylureas, e.g. tolbutamide and glibenclamide, are eliminated by the liver.

    (c) *False.* The effects and the risk of hypoglycaemia are particularly long-lasting in the elderly, mainly due to the decline in renal function and elimination of the drug.

    (d) *True.* This interaction side-effect is almost peculiar to chlorpropamide and can be reversed by naloxone.

    (e) *False.* This is a rare, but potentially lethal, side-effect of biguanides.

Renal
Questions

61 Frusemide:
   (a) Causes potassium retention.
   (b) Causes systemic alkalosis.
   (c) Is useful in the treatment of congestive heart failure.
   (d) Is often used in the long-term treatment of hypertension.
   (e) Has almost 100% bioavailability in cardiac failure.

62 Which of the following are physiological actions of angiotensin II?
   (a) Vasoconstriction.
   (b) Release of aldosterone.
   (c) Diuresis by a direct action on the kidney tubules.
   (d) Stimulation of thirst.
   (e) Alpha-adrenoceptor stimulation.

63 Thiazide diuretics:
   (a) May precipitate gout.
   (b) Are useful in the treatment of hypertension.
   (c) May precipitate diabetes mellitus.
   (d) May cause hypercalcaemia.
   (e) Inhibit sodium reabsorption in the distal convoluted tubules.

64 Which of the following statements about diuretics is/are correct?
   (a) Frusemide has its primary action on the loop of Henle, and gives a diuretic effect within a few minutes of intravenous administration.
   (b) Therapeutic drug level monitoring is useful.
   (c) Spironolactone antagonizes the effect of frusemide if the two drugs are used in combination.
   (d) Frusemide is a more potent antihypertensive agent than bendrofluazide.
   (e) Potassium supplements should always be given with thiazide diuretics.

65 Spironolactone:
   (a) Is a weaker diuretic than chlorothiazide.
   (b) Is a competitive aldosterone antagonist.
   (c) Is particularly useful in combination with angiotensin converting enzymes.
   (d) Has a slow onset but prolonged action.
   (e) Is well recognized as a precipitant of diabetes mellitus.

Renal

Answers

61 (a) *False.* Because frusemide prevents Na^+ reabsorption by the loop of Henle, distal tubular mechanisms act to reabsorb Na^+ in exchange for K^+ which is lost in the urine.

(b) *True.* Both H^+ and K^+ are lost into the urine in exchange for Na^+. The loss of H^+ results in an increase in HCO_3^- and produces a mild metabolic alkalosis with chronic therapy.

(c) *True.* To overcome the fluid retention.

(d) *False.* Once-daily frusemide is not as effective as once-daily thiazides for this condition.

(e) *False.* Frusemide's absorption is variable, typically about 60–75%, but this is further reduced in oedematous states, due to further impairment of absorption processes.

62 (a) *True.* It is a powerful vasoconstrictor.

(b) *True.* The renin–angiotensin system is a major regulator of aldosterone secretion.

(c) *False.* It has a Na^+-retaining effect, mediated via aldosterone's action on the tubules.

(d) *True.* It acts on the hypothalamus (outside of the blood–brain barrier).

(e) *False.* It has no direct effect on adrenoceptors. It may be involved in facilitating adrenergic mechanisms.

63 (a) *True.* But rare, by interfering with the tubular mechanisms for secreting uric acid, leading to urate retention and hyperuricaemia.

(b) *True.* The detailed mechanism is unknown. It reduces vascular responsiveness to constrictor influences, possibly as a result of subtle changes in intracellular Na^+ handling.

(c) *True.* But uncommon. Thought to be due to an effect on insulin release.

(d) *True.* But rare.

(e) *True.* At this site they can influence about 5% of total Na^+ reabsorption.

64 (a) *True.*

(b) *False.* The effect can be easily measured.

(c) *False.* This is a therapeutically useful combination with an additive diuretic effect and fewer side-effects. Spironolactone counters the stimulation of the renin–angiotensin–aldosterone system induced by frusemide.

(d) *False.* It is a more potent diuretic but, in single daily doses, probably as a result of a longer duration of action, the thiazide is a more effective antihypertensive drug.

(e) *False.* Thiazide and loop diuretics promote K^+ loss and there is an invariable small fall in serum K^+. In less than 10% of patients is this significant and requiring dietary supplementation.

65 (a) *True.* The potassium-sparing diuretics, which also include amiloride and triamterine, are weaker diuretics than the thiazides.

(b) *True.* It interferes with aldosterone's effect on the distal tubule and collecting ducts.

(c) *False.* The tendency to potassium retention which the ACE inhibitors produce could be dangerously exacerbated by concurrent spironolactone.

(d) *True.* As a diuretic it is generally thought to take two or three days before the effect of spironolactone is manifest.

(e) *False.* This is a feature of the thiazide group of diuretics and also of the loop diuretics.

Antimicrobials
Questions

66 In antimicrobial drug treatment:
- (a) Bactericidal drugs lead directly to the destruction of bacterial cells.
- (b) The ultimate efficacy of bacteriostatic drugs depends on the host's own defence mechanisms.
- (c) Antimicrobials produce their effect by interfering with metabolic pathways vital for the organism.
- (d) The production of an enzyme which destroys the antibacterial drug gives rise to one type of 'antibiotic resistance'.
- (e) The combination of a bactericidal and bacteriostatic drug is particularly efficacious.

67 The following observations about penicillins are correct:
- (a) They are bactericidal as a result of inhibition of bacterial cell wall synthesis.
- (b) They are widely distributed throughout the body including penetration even into normal CSF.
- (c) They are contraindicated in childhood and in pregnant women.
- (d) They are eliminated, in part, via the biliary tract.
- (e) They are well recognized as causing the side-effect of bone marrow suppression, particularly in infants.

68 Benzylpenicillin:
- (a) Can be effective when given orally to the elderly.
- (b) Is rapidly eliminated through the kidney.
- (c) Is usually administered parenterally.
- (d) Excretion may be reduced by probenecid.
- (e) Will cause a hypersensitivity reaction in persons known to have had a skin rash with ampicillin.

69 Within the penicillin group of antibiotics:
- (a) Ampicillin and flucloxacillin are suitable for oral administration.
- (b) Carbenicillin is a useful broad-spectrum antimicrobial drug.
- (c) Penicillinases act against the beta-lactam ring within the chemical structure of the penicillin.
- (d) Benzylpenicillin is particularly effective against Gram +ve organisms.
- (e) Allergic reactions are relatively common.

70 The cephalosporin group of antibiotics:
   (a) Have a beta-lactam ring, similar to that of the penicillins.
   (b) Generally are poorly absorbed from the GI tract.
   (c) Are mainly eliminated via the kidney.
   (d) Are the treatment of first choice when a broad-spectrum antibiotic is required in general practice.
   (e) Are ototoxic in patients with impaired renal function.

71 Sulphonamide antibacterial drugs:
   (a) Are eliminated both by the liver and by the kidney.
   (b) Are bacteriostatic.
   (c) Are recognized causes of photosensitive skin rashes.
   (d) Are particularly effective against pseudomonas species.
   (e) Interfere with the synthesis of folic acid.

72 Chloramphenicol:
   (a) Does penetrate the blood–brain barrier.
   (b) Must be administered parenterally.
   (c) Drug levels should be measured when used in premature infants.
   (d) Can cause depression of bone marrow function.
   (e) Causes discoloration of developing teeth when given to children.

73 Gentamicin:
   (a) Is eliminated by the kidney by glomerular filtration.
   (b) Is well absorbed from the GI tract.
   (c) Is an aminoglycoside antibiotic.
   (d) Has neuromuscular blocking activity.
   (e) Causes toxic damage to the eighth cranial nerve.

74 Rifampicin:
   (a) Is a potent enzyme inhibitor.
   (b) May cause an elevation in hepatic enzyme levels.
   (c) Is *only* effective against *Mycobacterium tuberculosis*.
   (d) Can interfere with the efficacy of the oral contraceptives.
   (e) Should be given in reduced dose to slow acetylators.

75 The following infections are correctly treated:
   (a) Severe, recurrent vaginal candidiasis by oral ketoconazole.
   (b) Oral 'thrush' (candidiasis) by topical nystatin.
   (c) Athlete's foot by amphotericin B.
   (d) Systemic fungal infections by griseofulvin.
   (e) Circumoral herpes simplex infections by acyclovir.

Antimicrobials
Answers

66 (a) *True.* By interfering with bacterial cell wall synthesis, intrabacterial protein synthesis, or folic acid production (a co-factor in nucleotide synthesis).

(b) *True.* The drug inhibits replication without destroying the organism.

(c) *True.* See (a).

(d) *True.* This is one major factor underlying antibiotic resistance, classically seen with penicillinase-producing organisms. The other major factor is the development of tolerance, i.e. the organism becomes able to grow despite the presence of the antibiotic.

(e) *False.* This combination is best avoided. Bactericidal drugs are most effective against replicating organisms. Replication is inhibited by bacteriostatic drugs.

67 (a) *True.*

(b) *False.* Although they are widely distributed they do not readily penetrate across the normal blood–brain barrier.

(c) *False.* In pregnancy and early childhood these drugs are relatively safe.

(d) *True.* The penicillin group undergoes enterohepatic recirculation with elimination from the body by renal mechanisms, by both glomerular filtration and tubular secretion.

(e) *False.* This side-effect is particularly associated with chloramphenicol.

68 (a) *False.*

(b) *True.* Elimination is by both glomerular filtration and active tubular secretion.

(c) *True.* Because of the problems of inactivation by gastric acid benzylpenicillin is usually administered parenterally.

(d) *True.* The elimination by active tubular secretion is blocked by probenecid. Thus higher blood levels of penicillin will be maintained for a longer period.

(e) *False.* The common skin rash associated with ampicillin is not always a true penicillin allergy. Nevertheless care should be taken in a patient who gives a previous history of skin rash with any penicillin.

69 (a) *True.* Ampicillin is a broad-spectrum penicillin and flucloxacillin is a penicillinase-resistant penicillin. Both are suitable for oral administration because they are relatively resistant to degradation by gastric acid. This resistance, however, is not absolute and both are destroyed to some extent, such that bioavailability is approximately 60%.

(b) *False.* Carbenicillin is the basic antipseudomonal penicillin.

(c) *True.* The alternative name for the penicillinases produced by bacteria is beta-lactamases.

(d) *True.* This is the major indication for benzylpenicillin and it is particularly potent against this type of organism.

(e) *True.* But these are usually mild and in only 0·1% of cases is there severe hypersensitivity.

70 (a) *True.* This in part explains their occasional cross-hypersensitivity reactions in patients known to be allergic to penicillins.

(b) *True.*

(c) *True.* They are similar to penicillins in that both glomerular filtration and active tubular secretion are involved in the renal elimination.

(d) *False.* They have no specific advantages and they are expensive.

(e) *False.* With the exception of occasional allergic reactions these drugs are well tolerated.

71 (a) *True.* Mainly by the kidney.

(b) *True.*

(c) *True.*

(d) *False.* They competitively inhibit the bacterial utilization of PABA.

(e) *True.* By interference with PABA.

72 (a) *False.* It is useful therapy in the treatment of meningitis due to *Haemophilus influenzae*.

(b) *False.* It is available for both oral and parenteral administration.

(c) *True.* Immature enzyme systems are unable adequately to metabolize the drug which thereby accumulates and can give rise to an adverse reaction characterized by cardiovascular collapse (the 'grey baby syndrome').

(d) *True.* Aplastic anaemia is a rare complication of chloramphenicol. It is partly an idiosyncratic reaction and partly dose-dependent.

(e) *False.* This is a complication of tetracycline therapy.

73 (a) *True.*   Therefore dosage adjustment is important if there is renal impairment.

   (b) *False.*   Oral absorption is negligible normally.

   (c) *True.*   As are streptomycin and neomycin.

   (d) *True.*   This is of little relevance under normal circumstances but may be important in patients with myasthenia gravis or in patients undergoing surgery who are receiving curare-like drugs.

   (e) *True.*   Both auditory and vestibular components may be affected.

74 (a) *True.*

   (b) *True.*   Particularly gamma-glutamyltranspeptidase.

   (c) *False.*   It is also useful, for example, against legionella species which cause legionnaires' disease.

   (d) *True.*   By enzyme induction.

   (e) *False.*   It does not undergo hepatic acetylation.

75 (a) *True.*   Ketoconazole is effective in various fungal conditions including mucocutaneous candidiasis. Its major side-effect is hepatotoxicity.

   (b) *True.*   Nystatin is effective for the topical treatment of yeast infections involving the skin and mucous membranes. It is not used parenterally because of the risks of toxicity.

   (c) *False.*   Although amphotericin B might be effective against athlete's foot (tinea pedis) the risk of adverse effects would contraindicate its use for such a trivial infestation. Adverse effects include nephrotoxicity.

   (d) *False.*   Griseofulvin is active only against dermatophytes in skin and nail infestations. It is administered orally. Systemic fungal infections require treatment with amphotericin B or flucytosine or miconazole.

   (e) *True.*   It is converted to the active metabolite by a herpes-coded enzyme.

Analgesics and Anti-inflammatory Drugs
Questions

76 Synthesis of prostaglandin:
- (a) Requires cyclo- and lipo-oxygenases.
- (b) Occurs in vesicles in a variety of cells throughout the body.
- (c) Is a part of the inflammatory response.
- (d) Is inhibited by non-steroidal anti-inflammatory drugs.
- (e) Is necessary for platelet aggregation.

77 Aspirin:
- (a) Reduces the normal body temperature.
- (b) Produces its analgesic effect primarily by altering perception of pain in the cerebral cortex.
- (c) Reduces platelet aggregation.
- (d) In high dose (5 g/day) is uricosuric.
- (e) Is excreted virtually unchanged by the kidney.

78 Indomethacin:
- (a) Is a non-steroidal anti-inflammatory drug.
- (b) Is an effective analgesic, even in the absence of acute inflammation.
- (c) Is a well-recognized cause of agranulocytosis.
- (d) Is highly bound to plasma protein.
- (e) Is relatively contraindicated during thiazide diuretic therapy.

79 An acute attack of gout:
- (a) Responds well to a combination of aspirin and probenecid.
- (b) Is best treated with allopurinol.
- (c) May be precipitated by treatment with uricosuric drugs, e.g. probenecid.
- (d) May be precipitated by diuretic treatment.
- (e) Typically responds within 48 hours to treatment with indomethacin.

80 Paracetamol:
- (a) Has clinically useful anti-inflammatory properties.
- (b) Has similar antipyretic activity to aspirin.
- (c) Is chemically related to phenacetin.
- (d) Is uricosuric.
- (e) Has a CNS component to its analgesic action.

81   Narcotic analgesics:
  (a) Act on specific opiate receptors in the CNS.
  (b) Stimulate receptors normally activated by endogenous opioids.
  (c) Have an euphoric effect.
  (d) Have a multiplicity of pharmacological effects.
  (e) Include morphine, heroin and codeine.

82   Which of the following may occur as a complication of morphine treatment of acute pain?
  (a) Addiction.
  (b) Antihistaminic effects.
  (c) A rise in systemic arterial blood pressure.
  (d) Constriction of smooth muscle sphincters.
  (e) Stimulation of the respiratory centre.

83   Morphine addicts typically show:
  (a) Tolerance to the CNS effects of morphine.
  (b) Pin-point pupils.
  (c) A withdrawal response following administration of naloxone.
  (d) Convulsions on withdrawal.
  (e) Cirrhosis of the liver.

84   Naloxone:
  (a) Is analgesic.
  (b) Causes euphoria.
  (c) Is the drug of first choice for the treatment of opiate overdose.
  (d) Is a partial agonist for the opiate receptor.
  (e) Induces a withdrawal syndrome if given to an opiate-dependent subject.

85   In the clinical management of pain:
  (a) Adequate analgesia is obtained with morphine only when it is intravenously administered.
  (b) Carbamazepine is useful in trigeminal neuralgia.
  (c) In chronic conditions, e.g. rheumatoid arthritis, methadone is an alternative to NSAIDs.
  (d) Diamorphine is less addictive than morphine.
  (e) Dihydrocodeine is less potent than codeine.

Analgesics and Anti-Inflammatory Drugs
Answers

76 (a) *True.*
    (b) *True.*
    (c) *True.*
    (d) *True.*
    (e) *True.*

77 (a) *False.* Aspirin's antipyretic activity is due to its antagonizing the effect on the hypothalamus of endogenous pyrogens from leucocytes.
    (b) *False.* It has a 'peripheral' analgesic action.
    (c) *True.* At *low* doses (<150 mg/day) it causes an irreversible inhibition of platelet cyclo-oxygenase and this leads to reduced production of thromboxane A_2 which is a potent platelet aggregator. (This selective effect on platelets is lost with higher doses.)
    (d) *True.* Inhibits proximal tubular reabsorption of urate.
    (e) *False.* Negligible amounts are excreted unchanged. Most is converted to salicylic acid by esterases in the liver and intestinal mucosa and then conjugated by the liver.

78 (a) *True.*
    (b) *False.* It is a potent anti-inflammatory drug with antipyretic activity but with modest analgesic effect.
    (c) *False.*
    (d) *True.* To albumin: as are most NSAIDs, though the binding may be saturable at high doses.
    (e) *True.* The effects of thiazides, particularly as anti-hypertensives, may be antagonized by indomethacin and other NSAIDs.

79 (a) *False.*   Although aspirin at high doses (> 3 g/day) has uricosuric
                      activity, <u>at usual doses it tends to cause urate retention
                      by interfering with distal tubular secretion</u>, and
                      additionally it antagonizes probenecid's effect on
                      proximal tubular reabsorption of water.

  (b) *False.*   Allopurinol is an xanthine oxidase inhibitor and thus
                 interferes with urate production, with increased levels of
                 the water-soluble hypoxanthine and xanthine, which are
                 both readily eliminated by the kidney.

  (c) *True.*   Thought to be due to mobilization of urate from tissue
                 deposits producing an inflammatory response.

  (d) *True.*   Thiazides and loop diuretics compete for urate transport
                 mechanisms in the renal tubule and thereby cause urate
                 retention.

  (e) *True.*   Also by other powerful non-steroidal anti-inflammatory
                 drugs. A similar rapid response may be achieved by
                 colchicine.

80 (a) *False.*   It is only a weak inhibitor of prostaglandin synthesis in
                      peripheral tissues.

  (b) *True.*

  (c) *True.*   Paracetamol is the major metabolite of phenacetin.

  (d) *False.*   In contrast to aspirin, it can be used in patients receiving
                 uricosuric drugs.

  (e) *True.*

81 (a) *True.*
  (b) *True.*
  (c) *True.*
  (d) *True.*
  (e) *True.*

82 (a) *False.*   Addiction is a complication of repeated administration
                      of morphine.

  (b) *False.*   As a rare side-effect, histamine release is promoted.

  (c) *False.*   A fall in systemic blood pressure is more usual.

  (d) *True.*

  (e) *False.*   Respiratory depression is a well-recognized hazard.

83 (a) *True.*   Thus the requirement for increasingly large doses.
  (b) *True.*
  (c) *True.*   By acute opiate antagonism.
  (d) *True.*
  (e) *False.*

84 (a) *False.*

(b) *False.*

(c) *True.*　Because it is a selective opiate antagonist and is free of agonist activity.

(d) *False.*　Partial agonist activity was a feature of its precursor, nalorphine.

(e) *True.*

85 (a) *False.*　Opiates are well absorbed from the GI tract (and from the nasal mucosa and lungs) and are effective: however, the intensity and duration of the analgesia varies accordingly to the route of administration.

(b) *True.*　It is especially useful for neuralgia, including trigeminal, tabetic and post-herpetic, but it has no general analgesic activity.

(c) *False.*　The risks of dependency and the relative lack of efficacy do not warrant treatment with opioids for chronic inflammatory diseases.

(d) *False.*　Both drugs have the same potential for addiction.

(e) *False.*　Dihydrocodeine is more potent.

Central Nervous System
Questions

86 Major tranquillizers:
(a) Are particularly useful as hypnotics.
(b) Include benzodiazepines.
——(c) Include phenothiazines and butyrophenones.
(d) Are used in the treatment of schizophrenia.
(e) Have dopamine antagonist properties.

87 Which of the following is/are true of chlorpromazine?
(a) It is antipsychotic because it stimulates dopamine receptors.
(b) It has alpha-adrenoceptor antagonist activity.
——(c) Its antiemetic activity is due solely to its anticholinergic activity.
(d) Hypothermia results from its action on the hypothalamus.
——(e) Jaundice of hepatocellular origin is a well-recognized side-effect.

88 The following statements about benzodiazepines are true:
(a) They do not reduce anxiety.
(b) They are used as hypnotics.
(c) They have anticonvulsant properties.
——(d) They are effective antidepressants.
(e) They are free of the risk of dependence.

89 Nitrazepam is considered a useful hypnotic because, under normal circumstances, it is free of the unwanted side-effects of:
(a) Addiction.
(b) Respiratory depression.
(c) 'Hangover'.
——(d) Increased CNS depression with ethyl alcohol.
(e) Disturbed sleep and nightmare on withdrawal.

90 Consider the following statements about benzodiazepines:
(a) Oral diazepam is a powerful anticonvulsant.
——(b) Temazepam is a long-acting benzodiazepine whose effects take up to one week to wear off.
——(c) Chlordiazepoxide suppresses unpleasant symptoms during alcohol withdrawal.
——(d) It is logical to use diazepam and nitrazepam together — as anxiolytic and hypnotic respectively.
(e) There is a recognized risk of respiratory arrest following intravenous diazepam.

91 The following drugs are useful as chronic therapy for grand mal epilepsy:
(a) Phenytoin.
(b) Carbamazepine.
(c) Chlormethiazole.
_(d) Diazepam.
(e) Chlorpromazine.

92 Tricyclic antidepressants:
(a) Include amitriptyline and imipramine.
—(b) Have a wide range of pharmacological properties including alpha-receptor antagonist activity, anticholinergic effects and non-specific sedative effects.
(c) Are extensively metabolized by the liver.
(d) Have the advantage of safety in overdosage.
_(e) Exert their antidepressant effects within 2–3 days of initiating treatment.

93 The following drugs are appropriate for the management of migraine:
(a) Ergotamine for infrequent minor attacks.
(b) Combination preparations with a simple analgesic and an antiemetic for relieving each acute attack.
(c) Pizotifen for long-term prophylaxis.
(d) High-dose clonidine for resistant cases.
(e) Methysergide in long-term low-dosage form for frequent mild attacks.

94 Levodopa diminishes the symptoms of Parkinsonism because:
(a) It is converted to dopamine in the CNS.
(b) There is a deficiency of dopamine in the brains of patients with this disease.
— (c) It blocks cholinergic receptors in the corpus striatum.
(d) It is converted to noradrenaline in sympathetic neurones.
—(e) It is an inhibitory transmitter.

95 Treatment of Parkinsonism with levodopa may:
(a) Reduce nausea and vomiting.
(b) Relieve rigidity.
—(c) Improve depression.
—(d) Induce mental illness.
(e) Cause hypertension.

Central Nervous System
Answers

86 (a) *False.* These drugs have a variety of effects on the CNS, including sedation, but they also alter cognitive, affective and motor function and accordingly are used in the treatment of psychoses.

(b) *False.* The benzodiazepines are minor tranquillizers, as is chlormethiazole.

(c) *True.* Phenothiazines (particularly chlorpromazine and fluphenazine), the butyrophenones (particularly haloperidol), and the thioxanthines (particularly flupenthixol) are all major tranquillizers.

(d) *True.* Chlorpromazine, fluphenazine and flupenthixol are particularly used in this condition.

(e) *True.* The phenothiazines act as dopamine receptor blockers hence their tendency to cause Parkinson-like syndromes.

87 (a) *False.* The precise mechanism of its antipsychotic activity is unknown. It acts as a dopamine antagonist and this is thought to be responsible for some of its side-effects.

(b) *True.* This is responsible for its side-effect of postural hypotension.

(c) *False.* There is a central component.

(d) *True.* This is a well-recognized complication, particularly of overdosage with phenothiazines generally.

(e) *False.* The jaundice attributable to chlorpromazine is an idiosyncratic cholestatic jaundice.

88 (a) *False.* The benzodiazepines act to reduce anxiety. Recent research suggests that there is a specific receptor in the brain upon which benzodiazepines act and thereby stimulate the inhibitory neurotransmitter, GABA.

    (b) *True.*

    (c) *True.* The anticonvulsant effect, however, is only obtained with very high plasma concentrations as are seen following intravenous bolus injection. Long-term oral therapy has no useful anticonvulsant effect.

    (d) *False.* The benzodiazepines are effective as anxiolytics, hypnotics and as general mild sedatives. They have no proven antidepressant activity.

    (e) *False.* It is now recognized that both psychological and physical dependency occurs with benzodiazepines and that there is an acute withdrawal (abstinence) syndrome.

89 (a) *False.* The benzodiazepine group is now generally recognized to be addictive.

    (b) *True.* Even in substantial overdosage respiratory depression does not occur if the drug is taken alone. However, benzodiazepines will potentiate the effect of other respiratory depressant drugs, including alcohol.

    (c) *False.*

    (d) *False.*

    (e) *True.* There is now a well-recognized withdrawal/abstinence syndrome.

90 (a) *False.* Intravenous diazepam has powerful anticonvulsant activity but oral diazepam does not produce sufficiently high plasma concentration.

    (b) *False.* Temazepam is a short-acting drug.

    (c) *True.*

    (d) *False.*

    (e) *True.*

91 (a) *True.*

    (b) *True.*

    (c) *False.* As with diazepam acute intravenous therapy with chlormethiazole is effective treatment for status epilepticus. However, long-term oral therapy does not have useful anticonvulsant activity.

    (d) *False.* As with chlormethiazole.

    (e) *False.* In fact chlorpromazine may worsen the tendency to seizures.

92 (a) *True.*
(b) *True.*   They competitively block the neuronal uptake of neurotransmitters, including noradrenaline and serotonin, and are thought to increase transmitter levels in the synaptic cleft. Additionally they alter the sensitivity of pre- and post-synaptic alpha-adrenoceptors and serotonin receptors and they have a general depressant effect on the CNS.
(c) *True.*   Some of the drugs in this group have active metabolites.
(d) *False.*   A major problem with tricyclic antidepressants is their potential for serious toxicity in overdosage, particularly cardiotoxicity and convulsions.
(e) *False.*   The therapeutic response to tricyclic antidepressants takes 2–3 weeks to develop.

93 (a) *False.*   Infrequent minor attacks are most appropriately treated with simple analgesic/antiemetic preparations. If attacks are severe, ergotamine preparations are indicated.
(b) *True.*
(c) *True.*   It is a serotonin antagonist and is used for the prophylaxis of frequent severe migraine.
(d) *False.*   Occasionally low-dosage clonidine (50–100 μg) is useful.
(e) *False.*   This serotonin antagonist was formerly used for prophylaxis, but the risk of serious adverse effects, particularly retroperitoneal fibrosis, has restricted its use to intermittent therapy for severe resistant cases.

94 (a) *True.*
(b) *True.*
(c) *False.*   L-Dopa has no anticholinergic activity.
(d) *True.*   The increase in noradrenergic mechanisms is thought to be responsible for some of the side-effects.
(e) *False.*

95 (a) *True.*
(b) *True.*
(c) *False.*
(d) *True.*
(e) *False.*   Postural hypotension is a more frequent side-effect.

Miscellaneous
Questions

96 In the management of medical conditions during pregnancy:
   (a) Warfarin should never be given in the first trimester.
   (b) Phenytoin plasma levels tend to fall during pregnancy.
   (c) Aspirin can safely be used except in the first trimester.
   (d) Ampicillin is teratogenic.
   (e) Chlorpropamide is useful in management of diabetes mellitus.

97 The following drugs are present in breast milk where they achieve clinically significant effects:
   (a) Cephalosporins.
   (b) Salicylates.
   (c) Benzodiazepines.
   (d) Narcotic analgesics.
   (e) Lithium.

98 The following treatments are recognized to be less effective in the elderly (over 70 years):
   (a) Atenolol for hypertension.
   (b) Digoxin for atrial fibrillation.
   (c) Indomethacin for rheumatoid disease.
   (d) Ipratropium (by inhalation) for chronic obstructive airways disease.
   (e) Temazepam for insomnia.

99 Which of the following drug-induced side-effect associations are recognized?
   (a) Haemorrhagic cystitis with cyclophosphamide.
   (b) Bone marrow suppression with doxorubicin.
   (c) Alopecia with etoposide.
   (d) Cardiomyopathy with cytarabine.
   (e) Nephrotoxicity with *cis*-platinum.

100 Which of the following cytotoxic agents are correctly categorized?
   (a) Methotrexate — antimetabolite.
   (b) 5-Fluorouracil — alkylating agent.
   (c) Doxorubicin (adriamycin) — antimetabolite.
   (d) Cyclophosphamide — alkylating agent.
   (e) Vincristine — antimitotic.

Miscellaneous
Answers

96 (a) *False.* Warfarin is a teratogen but women with prosthetic heart valves are at risk of thromboembolism if other anticoagulants are used.

    (b) *True.*

    (c) *False.* Aspirin at the end of pregnancy can cause haemostatic problems in the neonate.

    (d) *False.* The penicillins all appear to be safe.

    (e) *False.* It is possibly teratogenic and the necessary level of control requires insulin.

Note. As a general principle no drug should be considered absolutely safe in pregnancy, especially during the first trimester. Nevertheless, a number of drugs have been used sufficiently frequently during pregnancy to suggest that they are relatively free of teratogenic effects.

97 (a) *False.*

    (b) *False.*

    (c) *True.*

    (d) *True.*

    (e) *True.*

98 (a) *True.* Beta-adrenoceptor antagonists are less effective in the elderly.

    (b) *False.* There is a tendency for increased sensitivity to digoxin's effects, including an increased risk of side-effects.

    (c) *False.*

    (d) *False.* Tendency for increased efficacy.

    (e) *True.*

99 (a) *True.* The incidence of this complication, which is due to its metabolite acrolein, can be reduced if the specific antagonist mesna is co-administered.

(b) *True.* It shares the myelosuppressant properties of cytotoxic drugs generally.

(c) *True.* As a non-specific cytotoxic effect.

(d) *False.* This drug is a potent myelosuppressant (cardiotoxicity/cardiomyopathy is particularly associated with doxorubicin).

(e) *True.* *Cis*-platinum is generally toxic (myelotoxicity, ototoxicity, peripheral neuropathy) and also causes severe nausea and vomiting.

100 (a) *True.*

(b) *False.*

(c) *True.* To enalaprilic acid or enalaprilat.

(d) *True.* To prednisolone.

(e) *False.*

SECTION II

101 Jaundice is a well-recognized side-effect of:
(a) Halothane.
(b) Methyltestosterone.
(c) Propranolol.
(d) Ibuprofen.
(e) Prochlorperazine.

102 In clinical practice, morphine is particularly indicated for:
(a) Biliary colic.
(b) Gastrointestinal obstruction.
(c) Cardiac asthma (pulmonary oedema).
(d) Terminal cancer pain.
(e) Chronic respiratory disease.

103 Prolonged treatment with corticosteroids, e.g. prednisolone, causes:
(a) Dyspepsia.
(b) Osteomalacia.
(c) Hypertension.
(d) Diabetes mellitus.
(e) Thrombocytopenia.

104 The following drug combinations are potentially hazardous and are relatively contraindicated:
(a) 6-Mercaptopurine and allopurinol.
(b) Frusemide and gentamicin.
(c) Verapamil and atenolol.
(d) Indomethacin and carbenoxolone.
(e) Phenytoin and sodium valproate.

101 (a) *True.* Halothane causes hepatocellular necrosis.

(b) *True.* Other 17α-alkyl steroids (including the synthetic oestrogens of the 'pill') cause cholestasis without liver cell toxicity. There is probably a genetic predisposition.

(c) *False.* Propranolol is metabolized by the liver (first-pass effect) but does not cause liver damage.

(d) *False.*

(e) *True.* As do other phenothiazines, e.g. chlorpromazine.

102 (a) *False.* Pethidine is usually preferred because it does not produce an increased tone of the smooth muscle of the biliary tract, which may induce spasm and thereby worsen the colic and the pain.

(b) *False.* Morphine tends to reduce gastrointestinal motility.

(c) *True.* Both by its action to relieve the awareness of breathing and also because of its cardiac 'off-loading' effects due to pre-load reduction.

(d) *True.*

(e) *False.* The risks of respiratory depression are too great to warrant its use in chronic respiratory diseases.

103 (a) *True.* This is common. May be improved by enteric-coated tablets. The incidence of frank peptic ulceration is low.

(b) *False.* Osteoporosis may occur (but not osteomalacia, which is due to vitamin D deficiency).

(c) *True.* Related to sodium retention and increased vascular pressor responsiveness.

(d) *True.* Impaired carbohydrate tolerance is common.

(e) *False.* Corticosteroids tend to cause polycythaemia (they are often used to treat thrombocytopenia).

104 (a) *True.* Allopurinol inhibits the enzyme xanthine oxidase which is involved in the metabolism of 6-mercaptopurine: a dose reduction of 6-MCP is therefore required.

(b) *True.* An increased risk of nephrotoxicity has been reported.

(c) *True.* Both drugs have negative effects on cardiac conduction and contractility.

(d) *True.* Both may cause fluid retention.

(e) *False.* In fact may be useful because they have different antiepileptic activities.

105   The following statements about indomethacin are correct:
   (a)   Dizziness and lightheadedness are well-recognized side-effects.
   (b)   It has similar anti-inflammatory activity to paracetamol.
   (c)   Induces hepatic microsomal enzyme (mixed function oxidases) activity.
   (d)   Can usefully be combined with thiazide diuretics as anti-hypertensive therapy.
   (e)   Inhibits prostaglandin synthetase activity.

106   Insulin:
   (a)   Is a polypeptide.
   (b)   Is not suitable for human use if prepared from the bovine or porcine pancreas.
   (c)   Is effective if taken orally.
   (d)   Acts by enhancing cellular uptake of glucose.
   (e)   Acts by enhancing cellular utilization of glucose.

107   The kidney is an important route of excretion for:
   (a)   Atenolol.
   (b)   Acetylsalicylic acid.
   (c)   Pethidine.
   (d)   Diazepam.
   (e)   Chlorpropamide.

108   Phenytoin:
   (a)   Is eliminated exclusively according to first-order kinetics.
   (b)   Enhances its own metabolism during continued treatment.
   (c)   Is virtually free of toxic effects.
   (d)   Has the same plasma half-life at all doses and plasma concentrations.
   (e)   Is highly protein-bound.

109   Which of the following are true of digoxin therapy?
   (a)   The maintenance dosage depends largely on renal function.
   (b)   The half-life of digoxin is about 30 hours and so it can satisfactorily be administered once daily.
   (c)   Hypokalaemia protects the patient against digoxin toxicity.
   (d)   Toxicity can frequently first manifest as bradycardia.
   (e)   Phenytoin may be effective in digoxin-induced arrhythmias.

105 (a) *True.*   It is dose-related and occurs particularly in the elderly.
  (b) *False.* Paracetamol has no significant anti-inflammatory activity.
  (c) *False.*
  (d) *False.* Indomethacin's effects on the renal prostaglandin system may interfere with both the diuretic and antihypertensive effects of thiazide (and loop) diuretics.
  (e) *True.*   Like all non-steroidal anti-inflammatory drugs.

106 (a) *True.*   It is destroyed by gastrointestinal enzymes and therefore must be given parenterally.
  (b) *False.* Until recently bovine and porcine insulins were used. The incidence of sensitivity reactions was small.
  (c) *False.*
  (d) *True.*
  (e) *True.*

107 (a) *True.*   By glomerular filtration.
  (b) *True.*   Especially in alkaline urine.
  (c) *False.* Nomally only about 10%.
  (d) *False.* But its active metabolites, following hepatic metabolism, are renally excreted.
  (e) *True.*   Risk of prolonged hypoglycaemia in elderly patients with impaired renal function.

108 (a) *False.* At higher concentrations metabolism demonstrates zero-order kinetics.
  (b) *True.*   It induces hepatic microsomal enzyme activity.
  (c) *False.* High plasma concentrations are associated with cerebellar toxicity with ataxia, nystagmus, and diplopia.
  (d) *False.* The half-life at zero-order kinetics is significantly longer than the half-life at first-order kinetics.
  (e) *True.*   More than 90%.

109 (a) *True.*⎫ Digoxin is excreted primarily by glomerular filtration with a half-life of about 30 hours; renal impairment
  (b) *True.*⎭ is likely to lead to drug accumulation.
  (c) *False.* Hypokalaemia increases cardiac sensitivity to digoxin's effects.
  (d) *True.*   Bradycardia and ventricular ectopic activity, with 'coupled' beats, are characteristic.
  (e) *True.*   The anticonvulsant drug phenytoin has useful antidysrhythmic (class Ib) activity and is particularly useful in digoxin-induced dysrhythmias.

110 Hypersensitivity responses to penicillin:
- (a) May cause life-threatening anaphylactic shock.
- (b) Are more often of the delayed (IgM-mediated) type.
- (c) Usually disappear with repeated exposure to the drug.
- (d) Can be predicted reliably with skin testing.
- (e) Are more likely to occur if the patient is known to be allergic to cephalosporins.

111 Which of the following statements are correct?
- (a) Salbutamol has a greater cardiostimulant effect than isoprenaline.
- (b) Patients with obstructive airways disease are most appropriately treated with propranolol.
- (c) The hypotensive effect of atenolol is solely caused by reduction in cardiac output due to blockade of beta$_1$-adrenoceptors.
- (d) Propranolol is useful in the management of hyperthyroidism.
- (e) Of the range of available beta-blockers, atenolol is the most lipid-soluble and thus most likely to cause CNS side-effects.

112 Methysergide:
- (a) Rapidly aborts a migraine attack.
- (b) Precipitates angina pectoris in susceptible patients.
- (c) Causes retroperitoneal fibrosis during long-term therapy.
- (d) May be used to control symptoms in the carcinoid syndrome in which excess serotonin is produced.
- (e) Is chemically related to the hallucinogenic drug, LSD.

113 Which of the following may precipitate acute gout in susceptible individuals?
- (a) Thiazide diuretics.
- (b) Aminophylline.
- (c) Allopurinol.
- (d) Probenicid.
- (e) Colchicine.

110 (a) *True.* The incidence is very low: less than 0·05%.

(b) *True.* The delayed type is more common than the immediate type (which is IgE-mediated), with an overall incidence of about 5%. Skin rash is the most common manifestation.

(c) *False.*

(d) *False.* Skin testing is helpful but not absolutely reliable.

(e) *True.* Though the incidence of cross-hypersensitivity is low (10%).

111 (a) *False.* Salbutamol (and terbutaline) are both relatively selective for beta$_2$-adrenoceptors, i.e. non-cardiac.

(b) *False.* All beta-blockers should be avoided in obstructive airways disease but, if essential, metoprolol (and atenolol) are both more cardioselective than propranolol.

(c) *False.* The precise mechanism by which beta-blockers reduce blood pressure remains unclear: reduction in cardiac output is only one component in the long-term antihypertensive effect.

(d) *True.* The symptoms of hyperthyroidism reflect increased sensitivity of peripheral sympathetic activity.

(e) *False.* This description applies to propranolol: atenolol is water-soluble.

112 (a) *False.* It is used prophylactically, albeit rarely, for severe migraine.

(b) *True.* As a consequence of excessive vasconstriction.

(c) *True.* Continuous courses of therapy for more than 3–6 months are not recommended.

(d) *True.* Because of its serotonin antagonist effects.

(e) *True.* But it has no hallucinogenic properties.

113 (a) *True.* Interfere with (prevent) the tubular secretion of uric acid, thereby causing hyperuricaemia.

(b) *False.*

(c) *True.* ⎫ Both reduce serum urate in the long term but initially
              ⎬ may precipitate gout as a consequence of mobilization
(d) *True.* ⎭ of uric acid from tissue stores.

(e) *False.* Colchicine is used to treat acute gout.

114   In the treatment of Parkinson's disease:
   (a)   Benzhexol stimulates cholinergic receptors.
   (b)   Amantadine blocks cholinergic receptors.
   (c)   Salbutamol is particularly useful for controlling tremor.
   (d)   Chlorpromazine is relatively contraindicated.
   (e)   Decarboxylase inhibitors like carbidopa are useful because they
          have a selective action on the CNS.

115   The following statements are true:
   (a)   Atenolol is a selective beta$_2$-adrenoceptor antagonist.
   (b)   Bromocriptine is a serotonin antagonist.
   (c)   Salbutamol is a beta$_2$-adrenoceptor agonist.
   (d)   Chlorpromazine has alpha$_1$-adrenoceptor antagonist activity.
   (e)   Atropine is a beta-adrenoceptor agonist.

**116   The following drug combinations are recognized to have usefully
       additive therapeutic effects:**
   (a)   Trimethoprim and sulphamethoxazole.
   (b)   Nifedipine and metoprolol.
   (c)   Cimetidine and sucralfate.
   (d)   Frusemide and captopril.
   (e)   Lithium and bendrofluazide.

**117   The following drugs may cause convulsions in patients with no
       previous history of epilepsy:**
   (a)   Chlordiazepoxide.
   (b)   Disopyramide.
   (c)   Intravenous benzylpenicillin.
   (d)   Amitriptyline.
   (e)   Chlormethiazole.

118   Side-effects of chronic phenytoin therapy include:
   (a)   Cardiac dysrhythmias.
   (b)   Parkinsonian tremors.
   (c)   Loss of hair.
   (d)   Cerebellar dysfunction.
   (e)   Gingival hypertrophy.

114 (a) *False.* Benzhexol is an anticholinergic drug.

(b) *False.* This drug's mechanism of action is unclear. It appears to facilitate dopaminergic mechanisms.

(c) *False.* Salbutamol is a beta$_2$-adrenoceptor agonist which may cause tremor.

(d) *True.* Because it can cause a drug-induced Parkinsonian syndrome.

(e) *False.* Dopa decarboxylase inhibitors do not enter the CNS.

115 (a) *False.* It is preferentially a beta$_1$-adrenoceptor antagonist.

(b) *False.* It is a dopamine agonist.

(c) *True.*

(d) *True.* Although its activity is weak.

(e) *False.* It is anticholinergic.

116 (a) *True.* In a 1 to 5 ratio this forms the antibacterial drug co-trimoxazole.

(b) *True.* In the treatment of angina and hypertension.

(c) *False.* Sucralfate requires a highly acid pH to achieve optimal efficacy: the concurrent use of cimetidine significantly interferes with this.

(d) *True.* The antihypertensive effect of captopril is enhanced by concomitant diuretic therapy.

(e) *False.* Lithium reabsorption by the renal tubule is increased by diuretic therapy, with resultant high plasma levels and risk of CNS toxicity.

117 (a) *False.* Benzodiazepines have anticonvulsant activity.

(b) *True.* Particularly if high doses are given.

(c) *True.* If high doses are given and particularly if there is renal impairment.

(d) *True.* Especially in overdosage.

(e) *False.* It is a possible treatment for status epilepticus.

118 (a) *False.* Phenytoin has antiarrhythmic activity (class Ib).

(b) *False.*

(c) *False.* Growth of body hair is a complication of long-term phenytoin therapy, particularly in children.

(d) *True.* This is a manifestation of phenytoin toxicity, with nystagmus, ataxia and dysarthria.

(e) *True.* Particularly during long-term treatment in children.

119 **In salicylate poisoning:**
 (a) Depression of the respiratory centre is characteristic.
 (b) Hyperglycaemia is a recognized complication.
 (c) Severe metabolic acidosis is particularly common in children.
 (d) Treatment with forced alkaline diuresis may be effective.
 (e) Toxic symptoms correlate closely with the serum salicylate level.

120 **For angina pectoris, glyceryl trinitrate, which is taken sublingually:**
 (a) Is equally effective when given orally.
 (b) Often produces headache as a side-effect.
 (c) Causes a rise in intraocular pressure.
 (d) Causes a reduction in stroke volume of the heart.
 (e) May usefully be combined with a beta-adrenoceptor antagonist.

121 **The following drugs will achieve therapeutically effective plasma concentrations when taken orally, i.e. swallowed:**
 (a) Lignocaine.
 (b) Aminophylline.
 (c) Sodium aurothiomalate.
 (d) Insulin.
 (e) Cephalexin.

122 **The activity of the liver mixed function oxidase enzymes involved in drug metabolism:**
 (a) Is important for the metabolism for most water-soluble drugs.
 (b) Can be inhibited by cimetidine.
 (c) Can be induced by anticonvulsant drugs.
 (d) Can reduce the efficacy of the hormonal oral contraceptive agent.
 (e) Can be induced by rifampicin.

119 (a) *False.* Hyperventilation is characteristic.

  (b) *True.* Or hypoglycaemia: the disturbance of carbohydrate metabolism is variable.

  (c) *True.* Systemic acidosis is characteristic of poisoning in children: it is less often seen in adults.

  (d) *True.* Alkalinization of the urine is important for promoting pH-dependent component of elimination by the kidney.

  (e) *False.* There is only approximate correlation.

120 (a) *False.* There is considerable first-pass metabolism when taken orally, such that less then 10% of the ingested dose reaches the systemic circulation.

  (b) *True.* Related to dilatation of intracranial vessels.

  (c) *True.* Incipient glaucoma is a relative contraindication.

  (d) *True.* As a result of its venodilator activity with reduction in 'pre-load' to the right side of the heart.

  (e) *True.* To be taken intermittently as required, either in anticipation of an anginal attack or to abort it, whereas beta-blockers are taken on a regular basis as prophylaxis.

121 (a) *False.* Less than 10% bioavailable, as a result of extensive first-pass hepatic metabolism.

  (b) *True.* But aminophylline is a gastric irritant, leading to vomiting: 'slow-release' oral formulations and parenteral administration are preferred.

  (c) *False.* Not absorbed from the GI tract.

  (d) *False.* It is a peptide: destroyed in the GI tract by enzyme activity.

  (e) *True.* Although many other cephalosporins require parenteral administration.

122 (a) *False.* For many drugs, hepatic enzyme activity results in the production of water-soluble metabolites which are excreted by the kidney.

  (b) *True.* By a direct action to inhibit hepatic microsomal enzyme synthesis.

  (c) *True.* By phenytoin and phenobarbitone, and also by carbamazepine.

  (d) *True.* By promoting the breakdown of the constituent hormones.

  (e) *True.* Often detected in clinical practice by mild elevations of the hepatic enzyme gamma-glutamyltranspeptidase: this drug is also implicated in oral contraceptive failure.

123 **The following statements about non-steroidal anti-inflammatory drugs are true:**
(a) Aspirin is valuable in the treatment of gastrointestinal pain.
(b) Paracetamol is one of the most potent agents.
(c) Salicylates are effective in the treatment of rheumatoid arthritis.
(d) If administered parenterally the risk of gastric disturbance, particularly erosions and bleeding, is abolished.
(e) Aspirin has significant antipyretic activity.

124 **Acetylation in the liver is a major metabolic pathway for:**
(a) Hydralazine.
(b) Procainamide.
(c) Sulphasalazine.
(d) Dapsone.
(e) Isoniazid.

125 **The following drugs are used *orally* in the treatment of chronic stable angina. Their beneficial effect is thought to be due to:**
(a) Nifedipine — by reducing the work of the heart.
(b) Glyceryl trinitrate — by causing dilation of peripheral blood vessels.
(c) Metoprolol — by increasing sympathetic tone to the heart.
(d) Isosorbide dinitrate — by causing dilatation of the coronary arteries.
(e) Verapamil — by inhibiting the uptake of potassium by myocardial cells.

123 (a) *False.* Aspirin frequently causes gastric discomfort, dyspepsia and acute gastric erosions.

   (b) *False.* It has only weak anti-inflammatory activity.

   (c) *True.* They have effective analgesic and anti-inflammatory effects in this condition, but require to be taken in high doses, e.g. 2 g daily.

   (d) *False.* Prostaglandins are involved in gastric mucosal 'protection' and this will be affected even by systemic administration.

   (e) *True.* As also does paracetamol.

124 (a) *True.* Dosage restriction is recommended for slow acetylators.

   (b) *True.* The major metabolite, N-acetylprocainamide, is pharmacologically active with antidysrhythmic activity.

   (c) *True.* For the sulphapyridine moiety which is the absorbed component.

   (d) *True.*

   (e) *True.* Increased risk of peripheral neuropathy (pyridoxine-dependent) in slow acetylators and of hepatotoxicity in fast acetylators.

125 (a) *True.* At least part of the effect is due to a reduction in cardiac workload following peripheral arterial vasodilatation and after-load reduction.

   (b) *True.* The venodilator effect reduces the venous return to the heart (pre-load) and thus reduces cardiac workload.

   (c) *False.* It is a cardioselective beta-adrenoceptor antagonist which blocks the increases in the heart's oxygen requirements due to increased sympathetic activity.

   (d) *False.* Only with acute intravenous administration can an effect on coronary arteries be shown. Chronic oral nitrate therapy probably acts to reduce pre-load but whether or not it is useful in chronic angina remains in doubt.

   (e) *False.* It is a calcium channel blocker.

126   In the long-term treatment of grand mal epilepsy:
   (a)   Carbamazepine is effective.
   (b)   There is a direct and constant correlation between phenytoin plasma levels and the dose of the drug.
   (c)   Clonazepam is effective.
   (d)   In children, sodium valproate should *not* be prescribed.
   (e)   Phenobarbitone does *not* cause sedation.

127   Common unwanted effects of chlorpromazine include:
   (a)   Dystonic reactions.
   (b)   Hallucinations.
   (c)   Mood elevation.
   (d)   Anxiety.
   (e)   Jaundice.

128   The following statements about diuretics are correct:
   (a)   Mannitol exerts its main effect on the ascending limb of the loop of Henle.
   (b)   Chlorothiazide is useful additional treatment for gout.
   (c)   Loop diuretics have greater natriuretic potency than thiazide diuretics.
   (d)   Thiazide diuretics do not adversely affect the control of diabetes mellitus.
   (e)   Intravenous dopamine in low doses has a diuretic effect.

129   Constipation is often caused by:
   (a)   Atropine.
   (b)   Propranolol.
   (c)   Morphine.
   (d)   Magnesium trisilicate.
   (e)   Verapamil.

126 (a) *True.*   Probably now the drug of choice.

    (b) *False.* Although plasma levels can usefully be monitored and targeted for a therapeutic range, the pharmacokinetics of the drug are individual and complex, with zero-order kinetics at high doses.

    (c) *False.* Although this drug is effective acutely by intravenous administration for the relief of status epilepticus, it has little place as long-term oral therapy.

    (d) *False.* Sodium valproate may be useful in the management of grand mal epilepsy as well as of petit mal epilepsy.

    (e) *False.* Sedation is a well-recognized side-effect of phenobarbitone.

127 (a) *True.*   A variety of extrapyramidal syndromes have been observed. These are thought to be due to the drug's action as a dopamine receptor antagonist.

    (b) *True.*

    (c) *False.* It does not possess antidepressant activity; it may be used in the treatment of manic psychoses.

    (d) *False.*

    (e) *True.*   Characteristically a cholestatic jaundice.

128 (a) *False.* Mannitol is an osmotic diuretic. Following filtration by the glomeruli it is not absorbed to any extent from the tubular lumen and its osmotic effect prevents water reabsorption, particularly in the proximal tubule.

    (b) *False.* Thiazide diuretics interfere with tubular secretion of urate and may precipitate gout.

    (c) *True.*   Loop diuretics can affect about 15% of Na^+ reabsorption and thiazides about 5%.

    (d) *False.* Both thiazides and loop diuretics cause carbohydrate intolerance, perhaps by interfering with insulin secretion.

    (e) *True.*   Dopamine receptors in the kidney modulate renal blood flow and dopamine can thus increase glomerular filtration and urine production. Additionally there may be an increase in cardiac output. (At high doses, dopamine stimulates alpha-adrenoceptors and produces vasoconstriction.)

129 (a) *True.*   Anticholinergic action reduces gut motility.

    (b) *False.* Sympathetic blockade leaves unopposed cholinergic activity which may increase gut motility.

    (c) *True.*   Reduces peristalsis and increases sphincter tone.

    (d) *False.* Acts as an osmotic purgative.

    (e) *True.*   Interferes with the intracellular movement of calcium ions which are involved in gut motility.

130 The following statements about therapy with iron are true:
   (a) Parenteral administration produces a more rapid rise in haemoglobin than oral administration.
   (b) Desferrioxamine is useful in the treatment of overdosage with iron preparations.
   (c) Ascorbic acid impairs the efficiency of iron absorption.
   (d) Iron preparations should not be taken at the same time as tetracyclines.
   (e) Gastrointestinal side-effects often limit the use of oral iron preparations.

131 The combined hormonal oral contraceptive pill:
   (a) Increases the risk of ovarian carcinoma.
   (b) Inhibits ovulation.
   (c) Can precipitate migraine.
   (d) Can increase the incidence of venous thrombosis.
   (e) Should be avoided in women over 35 years who are cigarette smokers.

132 In the treatment of Parkinsonism:
   (a) Anticholinergic drugs should not be combined with levodopa.
   (b) Bromocriptine will antagonize the effects of levodopa.
   (c) Response to levodopa may be lost after several years.
   (d) Monoamine oxidase inhibitors may be useful.
   (e) Drug-induced Parkinsonism should be treated with levodopa.

133 Tricyclic antidepressants, such as imipramine:
   (a) Are free of adverse effects on the heart.
   (b) Can cause convulsions.
   (c) Exert an antidepressant effect within a few hours.
   (d) Can cause dry mouth and blurred vision.
   (e) Can cause postural hypotension.

130 (a) *False.* The rate of increase in haemoglobin is the same irrespective of the route of administration.

(b) *True.* It is a chelating agent. Administered orally it prevents iron absorption: parenterally, it forms complexes which are excreted in the urine.

(c) *False.* Acidity promotes the formation of ferrous ions (which are better absorbed) from ferric ions (which are the usual in food).

(d) *True.* Chelation occurs. The absorption of both is affected.

(e) *True.* Probably related to the dose of elemental iron and not significantly affected by the particular salt used.

131 (a) *False.* Ovarian and endometrial carcinoma is less common in 'pill' users.

(b) *True.* Due to feedback inhibition of FSH/LH secretion.

(c) *True.*

(d) *True.* Related to the oestrogen content. Less with oestrogen doses of less than 0·05 mg (or equivalent).

(e) *True.* The risk of cerebrovascular accident and myocardial infarction is significantly increased.

132 (a) *False.* This may be a useful combination because the anticholinergic drugs are most effective in controlling tremor whereas levodopa is most effective for hypokinesia and rigidity.

(b) *False.* In essence both drugs promote dopaminergic activity.

(c) *True.* There is a limited amount of evidence to suggest that the combined use of bromocriptine and levodopa might delay (*not* prevent) this development.

(d) *True.* Particularly the selective agents, e.g. selegiline.

(e) *False.* This type responds best to anticholinergic drugs.

133 (a) *False.* They cause serious tachydysrhythmias, as a result of both anticholinergic activity and facilitation of sympathetic tone (by blockade of noradrenaline re-uptake into neurones).

(b) *True.* Particularly in overdose, and particularly in children: probably related to the anticholinergic effects.

(c) *False.* The beneficial effects develop over a period of weeks.

(d) *True.* Anticholinergic side-effects also include constipation, urinary retention and tachycardia.

(e) *True.* Attributable to an alpha$_1$-adrenoceptor antagonist effect.

134 The diuretic chlorothiazide:
   (a) Is effective orally.
   (b) Causes potassium retention.
   (c) Antagonizes the action of digoxin.
   (d) Can aggravate diabetes mellitus.
   (e) Accelerates both sodium *and* chloride loss.

135 Which of the following statements are true?
   (a) Phenobarbitone can induce its own metabolism.
   (b) Primidone is metabolized to phenobarbitone.
   (c) Sodium valproate is effective only for the petit mal form of epilepsy.
   (d) Phenytoin can cause gum hyperplasia and acne.
   (e) Carbamazepine is used in the treatment of grand mal epilepsy.

136 Trimethoprim:
   (a) Acts by blocking ulilization of para-aminobenzoic acid (PABA).
   (b) Acts by inhibiting bacterial dihydrofolate reductase more than host dihydrofolate reductase.
   (c) Is bactericidal.
   (d) Is useful for the treatment of urinary tract infections.
   (e) Has a synergistic action when combined with a sulphonamide.

134 (a) *True.*   As are all of the thiazide diuretics.
    (b) *False.*   Potassium depletion and hypokalaemia are typical.
    (c) *False.*   There is no direct antagonism of the action of digoxin.
    (d) *True.*
    (e) *True.*

135 (a) *True.*   Phenobarbitone is a powerful inducer of the activity of the hepatic P450 enzyme system (mixed functional oxidases) which is responsible for its own metabolism and also the metabolism of a wide range of other drugs.
    (b) *True.*   Primidone is now little used because it offers no significant advantage over phenobarbitone, to which it is metabolized.
    (c) *False.*   Although initially developed for petit mal, valproate has also been shown to be effective in grand mal and in focal epilepsy.
    (d) *True.*   Chronic therapy in children is liable to cause gum hypertrophy, acne and hirsutism. Lymphadenopathy and skin rashes are rare complications of long-term therapy, as are vitamin D and folic acid deficiencies.
    (e) *True.*   Carbamazepine is used in the treatment of grand mal epilepsy and also of temporal lobe epilepsy. Carbamazepine and phenytoin are now the usual first-choice treatments for anticonvulsant therapy.

136 (a) *False.*   This is the mechanism of action of the sulphonamides.
    (b) *True.*
    (c) *False.*   Trimethoprim itself is bacteriostatic: the sulphonamide/trimethoprim combination is bactericidal.
    (d) *True.*
    (e) *True.*   See (c).

137 Drugs with H₁ histamine receptor antagonist properties:

(a) In therapeutic doses typically cause CNS stimulation with agitation and excitement.

(b) Are antiemetic.

(c) Include diphenhydramine.

(d) Interfere with allergic responses.

(e) Prevent histamine-induced gastric acid secretion.

138 Codeine:

(a) Is a constituent in opium.

(b) Frequently causes diarrhoea.

(c) Is used to treat nausea caused by morphine.

(d) Is equipotent with morphine.

(e) Depresses the cough reflex.

139 The following statements are true:

(a) Trimethoprim is useful for the treatment of urinary tract infections.

(b) Sulphonamides are excreted more rapidly when the urine is rendered alkaline.

(c) Hepatic acetylation is a major metabolic pathway for many of the sulphonamides.

(d) Co-trimoxazole is a combination of trimethoprim and sulphamethoxazole.

(e) Sulphasalazine is useful therapy for ulcerative colitis.

137 (a) *False.*   In therapeutic doses general CNS depression and somnolence are customary. In overdosage restlessness and insomnia and fits may occur.

(b) *True.*   Particularly the treatment of motion sickness.

(c) *True.*   Also chlorpheniramine, cyclizine, promethazine and the newer agents, including terfenadine and astemizole, which seem less likely to cause sedation and psychomotor impairment.

(d) *True.*   Histamine is the mediator of the allergic response and these drugs prevent histamine acting on its receptor sites. Antihistamine drugs do not prevent the release of histamine.

(e) *False.*   Gastric acid secretion is dependent upon the stimulation of the H_2-receptor. Conventional antihistamine drugs do not act upon the H_2-receptor.

138 (a) *True.*   Opium contains numerous alkaloids of which morphine, codeine and papaverine have clinical usefulness.

(b) *False.*   Its most frequent use is as an antidiarrhoeal agent because of its peripheral effect on reducing motility and secretion within the gastrointestinal tract.

(c) *False.*   Although its central effects are much weaker than those of morphine, its actions are similar and therefore it would tend to promote nausea.

(d) *False.*   It has less than 1/10th the potency of morphine.

(e) *True.*   This is its other major therapeutic indication.

139 (a) *True.*   It is as effective as the combination preparation, co-trimoxazole.

(b) *True.*   Generally the solubility (degree of ionization) of the sulphonamides is increased at higher pH.

(c) *True.*   In fact, sulphadimidine may be used as a test of acetylator status.

(d) *True.*   It contains sulphamethoxazole and trimethoprim in the ratio of 5:1.

(e) *True.*   Sulphasalazine is a combination of 5-aminosalicylic acid (which is poorly absorbed from the GI tract) and sulphapyridine.

140 **Which of the following drugs have pharmacologically active metabolites?**
(a) Cyclophosphamide.
(b) Procainamide.
(c) Levodopa.
(d) Prednisone.
(e) Enalapril.

141 **Which of the following are common results of treatment with cytotoxic drugs?**
(a) Immunosuppression.
(b) Alopecia.
(c) Renal failure.
(d) Thrombocytopenia.
(e) Leucopenia.

142 **If warfarin is given to a patient who has been habitually taking a barbiturate hypnotic:**
(a) The barbiturate dose will have to be increased to produce the same effect.
(b) The warfarin will have to be given in bigger than usual doses.
(c) The patient will bleed excessively following trivial injury.
(d) Warfarin will have greater activity because it is displaced from binding sites on circulating plasma protein.
(e) The rate of metabolism of warfarin is slower than normal.

143 **Body weight gain may occur following the clinical use of which of the following drugs?**
(a) Carbenoxolone.
(b) Combined progesterone/oestrogen contraceptives.
(c) Nifedipine.
(d) Bendrofluazide.
(e) Fenfluramine.

140 (a) *True.* Both 4-hydroxycyclophosphamide and aldophosph-
amide are active metabolities.

(b) *True.* N-acetyl procainamide is an active metabolite.

(c) *True.* Dopa decarboxylase in the CNS metabolizes L-dopa to
the neurotransmitter dopamine.

(d) *True.* It is metabolized to the active form, prednisolone.

(e) *True.* It is de-esterified primarily in the liver to the active
form, enalaprilic acid.

141 (a) *True.*

(b) *True.*

(c) *True.*

(d) *True.*

(e) *True.*

142 (a) *False.* Warfarin does not affect the disposition of barbiturates.

(b) *True.* Because the hepatic enzyme activity will have already
been induced by the barbiturate.

(c) *False.* The opposite trend will apply.

(d) *False.*

(e) *False.*

143 (a) *True.* Due to an aldosterone-like effect leading to salt and
water retention.

(b) *True.* An aldosterone-like effect.

(c) *True.* Dihydropyridine calcium antagonists may cause
peripheral oedema with or without a change in body
weight.

(d) *False.*

(e) *False.* This is an amphetamine derivative which has appetite
suppressant activity.

144 **Hypertension is a recognized complication of therapeutic doses of:**
(a) Tricyclic antidepressants.
(b) Combined hormonal oral contraceptives.
(c) Anti-inflammatory corticosteroids.
(d) Salicylates.
(e) Beta-adrenoceptor antagonists.

145 **Impaired renal function is a recognized adverse effect of:**
(a) Penicillamine.
(b) Allopurinol.
(c) Sodium aurothiomalate.
(d) Glyceryl trinitrate.
(e) Daunorubicin.

146 **Dextropropoxyphene:**
(a) Is chemically related to methadone.
(b) Has similar analgesic potency to pethidine.
(c) Is a weak inhibitor of hepatic mixed function oxidases.
(d) In overdose causes death due to hepatotoxicity.
(e) Is not addictive.

144 (a) *False.* In clinical practice a fall in blood pressure is usually seen, probably as a result of peripheral alpha-adrenoceptor antagonism. In the CNS these drugs block neurotransmitter re-uptake mechanisms. In the periphery this mechanism might be expected to facilitate vasoconstriction.

(b) *True.* Only about 5% of women have an increase in blood pressure which might be classified as hypertension. The mechanism relates to altered sodium homeostasis and enhanced vasoconstrictor responsiveness, primarily due to oestrogen.

(c) *True.* Due mainly to Na^+ retention and to increased pressor responsiveness.

(d) *False.* Although drugs with prostaglandin synthetase effects may interfere with the action of antihypertensive drugs, especially diuretics, there is no evidence that salicylates themselves increase blood pressure.

(e) *False.* Blockade of peripheral vascular beta-receptors promotes vasoconstriction: however, the overall effect of systemic beta-blockade is a fall in blood pressure.

145 (a) *True.* Proteinuria: which may be sufficiently severe to produce the nephrotic syndrome. Probably due to an immune complex nephritis.

(b) *False.* Allopurinol is an xanthine oxidase inhibitor. In contrast to uricosuric drugs it has no effect on tubular function.

(c) *True.* Probably a direct 'toxic' effect on the proximal tubule, leading to proteinuria, and sometimes nephrosis.

(d) *False.* Undergoes rapid presystemic metabolism and there is no recognized metabolite nephrotoxicity.

(e) *False.* Cardiotoxicity, not nephrotoxicity, is a well-recognized complication of this anticancer drug.

146 (a) *True.*

(b) *False.* It has only weak analgesic properties.

(c) *True.*

(d) *False.* The risk from dextropropoxyphene is respiratory depression. Hepatic damage is a feature of poisoning with paracetamol with which it is often combined in proprietary analgesic combinations.

(e) *False.*

147 **Neutropenia and agranulocytosis are recognized hazards of:**
(a) Long-term corticosteroid therapy.
(b) Treating chronic inflammatory conditions with ibuprofen.
(c) Chloramphenicol.
(d) Gold salts for rheumatoid arthritis.
(e) 5-Fluorouracil.

148 **Beta-adrenoceptor antagonists are useful in the management of:**
(a) Heart failure.
(b) Bronchial asthma.
(c) Angina pectoris.
(d) Intermittent claudication.
(e) Thyrotoxicosis.

149 **Morphine:**
(a) Is a metabolite of codeine.
(b) Typically causes vomiting.
(c) Typically causes diarrhoea.
(d) Has specific receptors in the CNS.
(e) Has specific receptors in the gastrointestinal tract.

150 **Which of the following cytotoxic drugs is/are classified as antimetabolite(s)?**
(a) Azathioprine.
(b) Vincristine.
(c) Methotrexate.
(d) Cyclophosphamide.
(e) Cortisol.

147 (a) *False.* There is an antilymphocyte effect but usually an increase in the number of granulocytes.

(b) *False.* Ibuprofen has not been implicated but phenylbutazone has.

(c) *True.* A dose-related leucopenia occurs and aplastic anaemia has also been reported, probably as a sensitivity reaction.

(d) *True.* A toxic effect on the bone marrow.

(e) *True.* As an expected result of its cytotoxic action.

148 (a) *False.* In this situation there is increased adrenergic drive trying to compensate for the failing heart. Blockade of this drive may worsen (or precipitate) cardiac failure.

(b) *False.* Increased sympathetic activity at the bronchial $beta_2$-receptor opposes bronchoconstriction in bronchial asthma: if the $beta_2$-receptor is blocked asthma will be worsened, or precipitated.

(c) *True.* Due to reduction of the myocardial oxygen demand both by attenuating the heart rate increase which normally accompanies exercise and also by a direct, and undefined, action on the myocardium.

(d) *False.* Beta-blockers impair $beta_2$-receptor-mediated vaso-dilatation in skeletal muscle and also tend to reduce cardiac output.

(e) *True.* There is increased sensitivity to catecholamines. Symptoms, both peripheral (tremor) and cardiac (tachycardia), are improved by beta-blockers.

149 (a) *True.*

(b) *True.*

(c) *False.*

(d) *True.*

(e) *True.*

150 (a) *True.* Via its active metabolite, 6-mercaptopurine, which inhibits DNA synthesis.

(b) *False.*

(c) *True.* By inhibiting folic acid metabolism.

(d) *False.* It is an alkylating agent.

(e) *False.* This is used as adjuvant cytotoxic therapy on account of its effect against lymphoid cells and tissues.

151 In the clinical management of migraine:
- (a) Pizotifen is used prophylactically.
- (b) Ergotamine powder may be administered by aerosol inhaler.
- (c) Aspirin is of value in mild attacks.
- (d) Headache may be a side-effect of ergotamine.
- (e) The hormonal contraceptive pill increases the frequency of attacks in some women.

152 Recognized adverse effects of hydralazine include:
- (a) Impotence.
- (b) Lupus erythematosus syndrome.
- (c) Tachycardia.
- (d) Constipation.
- (e) Difficulty in accommodating for near vision.

153 Which of the following drugs is of established value in the treatment of stable angina pectoris?
- (a) Verapamil.
- (b) Flecainide.
- (c) Propranolol.
- (d) Salbutamol.
- (e) Digoxin.

154 In the treatment of rheumatoid arthritis:
- (a) Headache is a recognized side-effect of indomethacin.
- (b) A single intramuscular injection of sodium aurothiomalate is almost completely removed from the body within 48 hours.
- (c) Mefenamic acid is free of adverse gastrointestinal effects.
- (d) Ibuprofen inhibits the activity of prostaglandin synthetase.
- (e) There is a risk of adrenal insufficiency with long-term prednisolone.

151 (a) *True.*   Vasoconstriction following serotonin release has been implicated in the cause of migraine: pizotifen has serotonin antagonist activity.

(b) *True.*   Oral absorption is poor and often further complicated by the gastric atony and vomiting which occur in migraine.

(c) *True.*   Mild attacks may respond to simple analgesia, sometimes combined with an antiemetic.

(d) *True.*   Probably due to excessive and prolonged vasoconstriction.

(e) *True.*

152 (a) *False.*   Hydralazine is a 'direct' vasodilator which does not interfere with sympathetic or parasympathetic function.

(b) *True.*   This is a dose-related effect, commoner in slow acetylators.

(c) *True.*   Tachycardia and palpitations, which result from reflex sympathetic activation, are often symptomatic.

(d) *False.*

(e) *False.*

153 (a) *True.*   A calcium channel blocker.

(b) *False.*   A class I antidysrhythmic.

(c) *True.*   A beta-adrenoceptor antagonist (non-selective).

(d) *False.*   A beta$_2$-adrenoceptor agonist.

(e) *False.*   A cardiac glycoside.

154 (a) *True.*   Headache and lightheadedness occur in 10–20% of patients initially, especially if high doses are used.

(b) *False.*   Only 5–10% is eliminated. Gold salts are strongly bound to tissue proteins and accumulation occurs, particularly in liver, spleen and kidney.

(c) *False.*   All NSAIDs are liable to cause gastric disturbance, probably because gastric mucosal protection depends on prostaglandins.

(d) *True.*   Inhibition of prostaglandin synthesis, and thereby of the inflammatory response, seems to be the main therapeutic action of all NSAIDs.

(e) *True.*   Due to suppression by the exogenous steroid of pituitary release of ACTH. The lack of ACTH leads to atrophy of the adrenal gland.

155 Verapamil:
- (a) May be used to treat atrial arrhythmias.
- (b) Frequently causes constipation.
- (c) Should not be used in asthmatic patients.
- (d) Blocks slow calcium channels in smooth muscle.
- (e) Is often given with beta-blockers in hypertension.

156 Because of a potentially undesirable interaction aspirin is contraindicated in patients already receiving:
- (a) Digoxin.
- (b) Warfarin.
- (c) Benzodiazepines.
- (d) Dipyridamole.
- (e) Probenecid.

157 The antiparkinsonian drug levodopa:
- (a) Has useful antihypertensive activity.
- (b) Is best combined with a dopa decarboxylase inhibitor to reduce metabolic degradation.
- (c) Is converted to a false transmitter.
- (d) Can precipitate psychiatric disturbances.
- (e) Is actively taken up by dopaminergic neurones in the CNS.

155 (a) *True.*

(b) *True.* This is one of the commonest side-effects.

(c) *False.* Verapamil can safely be used in the asthmatic patient with angina or hypertension and may indeed have some weak bronchodilator action in its own right.

(d) *True.* It also blocks certain channels in cardiac but not skeletal muscle.

(e) *False.* Because of combined negative chronotropic and inotropic effects this combination is only rarely used.

156 (a) *False.*

(b) *True.* As a result of competition for protein binding sites there is an increased amount of 'free' warfarin and thereby an enhanced anticoagulant effect. Additionally, the consequences of gastric erosions and bleeding are potentially more serious in an anti-coagulated patient.

(c) *False.*

(d) *False.* Although there is limited evidence of a useful additive effect these drugs are often combined as antiplatelet therapy.

(e) *True.* Probenecid exerts its uricosuric effect by interfering with the organic acid re-uptake mechanisms in the renal tubule: salicylates compete with this, particularly at high doses.

157 (a) *False.* The effect on blood pressure is unpredictable and variable with a tendency to cause symptomatic postural hypotension.

(b) *True.* Carbidopa and benserazide are dopa decarboxylase inhibitors which do not cross the blood–brain barrier but act peripherally to prevent degradation of L-dopa.

(c) *False.* L-dopa is converted in the brain to the neurotransmitter dopamine.

(d) *True.* The formation of dopamine and other catecholamines within the central nervous system may precipitate various psychoses, including manic depression.

(e) *True.*

158 **Terfenadine, a selective H₁ antagonist:**
- (a) Will cause more sedation than diphenhydramine.
- (b) Will heal 80% of duodenal ulcers in six weeks.
- (c) May control symptoms of hay fever.
- (d) Can cause physical dependence and addiction.
- (e) May improve symptoms in chronic bronchitis.

159 **Frusemide:**
- (a) Is a weaker diuretic than chlorothiazide.
- (b) Has its main effect on the distal convoluted tubule.
- (c) Is short-acting.
- (d) Is effective orally.
- (e) Is effective, in high doses, in renal failure.

160 **The following drugs control cardiac dysrhythmias in clinical practice by the mechanism indicated:**
- (a) Lignocaine decreases the rate of rapid depolarization of cardiac cells.
- (b) Propranolol has potent membrane stabilizing activity.
- (c) Verapamil has beta-adrenoceptor antagonist properties.
- (d) Digoxin decreases atrioventricular conduction.
- (e) Amiodarone prolongs the refractory period of the cardiac action potential.

158 (a) *False.* The newer antihistamine drugs, terfenadine and astemizole, cross the blood–brain barrier much less readily than the earlier type. Thus, sedation, psycho-motor impairment and alcohol potentiation are less problematical.

(b) *False.* Ulcer healing, as a result of reduced gastric acid secretion, relates to the H_2-receptor antagonist drugs, e.g. cimetidine, ranitidine.

(c) *True.* The antiallergic properties depend on antagonism of H_1-mediated effects.

(d) *False.*

(e) *False.* This disorder does not have an allergic component.

159 (a) *False.* Both frusemide and bumetanide, which are loop diuretics, have more powerful natriuretic and diuretic activity than the thiazides.

(b) *False.* Its major effect is on the ascending limb of the loop of Henle.

(c) *True.* Following oral administration the onset of action is typically within 30–60 minutes and the diuretic effect is complete by about six hours.

(d) *True.*

(e) *True.* In contrast to the thiazides which lose their efficacy when the GFR falls to less than 25 ml/min: 10 times the usual doses may be required.

160 (a) *True.* The threshold for depolarization is increased and the rate of depolarization is decreased (class Ia).

(b) *False.* This property is not relevant at the plasma concen-trations achieved clinically. Its antidysrhythmic effect is related to its beta-adrenergic effects: thus, it is useful in supraventricular tachydysrhythmias.

(c) *False.* It is a calcium channel blocker.

(d) *True.*

(e) *True.*

161 **Which of the following drugs increase the urinary excretion of uric acid?**
(a) Low doses (less than 300 mg daily) of aspirin.
(b) Allopurinol.
(c) Sulphinpyrazone.
(d) Frusemide.
(e) Probenecid.

162 **Parkinsonism may be aggravated by:**
(a) Promethazine.
(b) Haloperidol.
(c) Anticholinesterase drugs.
(d) Diazepam.
(e) Bromocriptine.

163 **Which of the following is/are appropriate long-term treatments for petit mal and myoclonic/clonic seizures in childhood?**
(a) Amphetamine.
(b) Carbamazepine.
(c) Metoclopramide.
(d) Sodium valproate.
(e) Clonazepam.

164 **Glyceryl trinitrate:**
(a) Is the treatment of choice in congestive heart failure.
(b) Has to be metabolized to a dinitrate before it is effective.
(c) Has a duration of action of several hours following buccal absorption.
(d) Can cause a fall in blood pressure.
(e) Can increase exercise tolerance if taken immediately before exercise.

165 **Beta-adrenoceptor antagonists:**
(a) Tend to lose their selectivity for the beta$_1$-receptors as dosage is increased.
(b) Are relatively contraindicated in peripheral vascular disease.
(c) Are drugs of choice in the treatment of variant (Prinzmetal's) angina.
(d) If hydrophilic are more likely to cause central nervous system disturbance.
(e) Frequently cause postural hypotension.

161 (a) *False.* Interference with renal tubular reabsorption of urate only occurs with high-dose salicylates.

(b) *False.* Allopurinol reduces uric acid concentrations by inhibiting the enzyme xanthine oxidase, thereby preventing the formation of uric acids.

(c) *True.* Both sulphinpyrazone and probenecid are classified as uricosuric drugs: they promote the loss of uric acid by inhibiting the reabsorption of urate by the renal tubules.

(d) *False.* Like thiazide diuretics, it may cause urate retention.

(e) *True.*

162 (a) *True.* As a consequence of its effects as a dopamine receptor antagonist.

(b) *True.* As above.

(c) *True.* Effectively these drugs enhance cholinergic activity.

(d) *False.*

(e) *False.* This drug has a limited therapeutic role in the treatment of Parkinson's disease.

163 (a) *False.* This drug was used as an appetite suppressant: it is now obsolete.

(b) *False.* The incidence of side-effects outweighs its potential benefit.

(c) *False.* This is an antiemetic.

(d) *True.* This is the drug of choice.

(e) *True.* Though more sedative than valproate.

164 (a) *False.* Its duration of action is too short.

(b) *False.*

(c) *False.* Its effects last only a few minutes.

(d) *True.* It relaxes peripheral vascular smooth muscle, venular more than arteriolar.

(e) *True.* By reducing cardiac pre-load.

165 (a) *True.* Selectivity is relative: it is most apparent at low doses.

(b) *True.* By permitting unopposed alpha-adrenoceptor-mediated constriction of peripheral blood vessels.

(c) *False.* This syndrome is thought to be due to coronary artery spasm which may be worsened by beta-blockade (because of unopposed alpha-adrenoceptor tone in the coronary arteries).

(d) *False.* It is the lipophilic type, particularly propranolol, which crosses the blood–brain barrier.

(e) *False.*

166   Glucocorticoids are clinically useful in the treatment of:
(a)   Peptic ulcer.
(b)   Ulcerative colitis.
(c)   Acute leukaemia in children.
(d)   Acute psychosis.
(e)   Cushing's disease.

167   Chlorpromazine:
(a)   Is indicated in the treatment of epilepsy.
(b)   May cause Parkinsonism.
(c)   Can produce cholestatic jaundice.
(d)   Can upset temperature regulation.
(e)   Is useful in the treatment of diabetes mellitus.

168   Which of the following statements about the narcotic analgesics is/are correct?
(a)   Codeine has useful antitussive properties.
(b)   Codeine has useful antipyretic properties.
(c)   Heroin is less addictive than morphine.
(d)   Pentazocine may cause hallucinations.
(e)   Diamorphine is used to control severe diarrhoea.

169   The following drugs should be avoided or used at reduced dosage in patients who have impaired renal function:
(a)   Captopril.
(b)   Digoxin.
(c)   Lignocaine.
(d)   Gentamicin.
(e)   *Cis*-platinum.

166 (a) *False.*   Steroids delay ulcer healing and may precipitate gastric bleeding.

   (b) *True.*   Systemic steroid therapy is reserved for severe cases but topical steroid therapy, in the form of suppositories or enemata, is frequently used for localized disease of the lower large intestine.

   (c) *True.*   Steroids are useful adjuvant therapy because of their antilymphocytic effects.

   (d) *False.*   Overt psychosis of the manic depressive form is a recognized complication of high-dose steroid therapy.

   (e) *False.*   Cushing's disease results from excessive natural production of glucocorticoids.

167 (a) *False.*   It has a tendency to worsen epilepsy.

   (b) *True.*   As a result of its dopamine receptor-blocking effect in the brain.

   (c) *True.*   This is a well-recognized hypersensitivity effect.

   (d) *True.*   Typically leading to hypothermia.

   (e) *False.*   Chlorpromazine is one of the phenothiazine group of drugs: chlorpropamide is one of the sulphonylurea group which is used in diabetes.

168 (a) *True.*   This is one of its major uses.

   (b) *False.*   It has no antipyretic activity.

   (c) *False.*   They are comparable.

   (d) *True.*   Particularly in the elderly.

   (e) *False.*   Codeine is useful for this purpose and does not carry the same hazards of addiction and respiratory depression.

169 (a) *True.*   Increased risk of further impairment of renal function.

   (b) *True.*   It is 60–90% eliminated by the kidney and may accumulate in renal failure.

   (c) *False.*   It is extensively metabolized by the liver.

   (d) *True.*   It is eliminated primarily by glomerular filtration. Additionally the risk of nephrotoxicity appears to be greater if there is previous renal damage.

   (e) *True.*

170 Ergotamine is:
(a) A peripheral vasoconstrictor.
(b) Recommended for long-term prophylaxis against severe migraine.
(c) A weak alpha-adrenoceptor blocker.
(d) Useful in the treatment of migraine.
(e) A 5-hydroxytryptamine (5-HT) antagonist.

171 The following are known complications of thiazide diuretic therapy:
(a) Thrombocytopenia.
(b) Hyperkalaemia.
(c) Gynaecomastia.
(d) Hyperuricaemia.
(e) Peptic ulceration.

172 In hyperthyroidism:
(a) Beta-blockers reduce the circulating levels of thyroid hormone.
(b) Carbimazole exerts its effect within 24–48 hours.
(c) Lithium may exacerbate the symptoms.
(d) Agranulocytosis is an important adverse effect of carbimazole.
(e) Radioiodine is the treatment of choice in young patients (under 40 years).

173 Long-term administration of prednisolone in humans characteristically causes:
(a) Increased secretion of adrenocorticotrophic hormone (ACTH).
(b) A reduced rate of wound healing.
(c) Lowered resistance to infection.
(d) Hypertension.
(e) Suppression of antibody synthesis.

174 In the treatment of iron deficiency anaemia:
(a) Ferrous sulphate is the preferred treatment.
(b) Giving iron alone may precipitate subacute combined degeneration.
(c) The dose of parenteral iron should be related to initial haemoglobin concentration.
(d) Treatment is only necessary until the anaemia is corrected.
(e) Diarrhoea is a dose-related effect.

170 (a) *True.*   It is a powerful direct vasoconstrictor (it has weak, alpha-blocking activity also).

(b) *False.*   It is reserved for acute attacks of migraine: the toxic effects of irreversible vasoconstriction may occur with continued administration.

(c) *True.*   See (a).

(d) *True.*   Probably by causing vasoconstriction and thereby reducing the amplitude of the changes in vascular tone. Platelet factors have also been complicated in migraine and these may be affected by ergotamine's alpha and serotonin antagonist effects.

(e) *True.*   It is chemically related to methysergide and both drugs inhibit the actions of serotonin.

171 (a) *True.*   Well recognized, but rare and usually reversible.

(b) *False.*   Both thiazide and loop diuretics cause a fall in serum potassium.

(c) *False.*   This is a side-effect of the potassium-sparing diuretic, spironolactone, which has a steroid structure.

(d) *True.*   And, rarely, gout may be precipitated in susceptible individuals.

(e) *False.*

172 (a) *False.*   Beta-adrenoceptor blockers provide symptomatic improvement by interfering with the action of thyroid hormones.

(b) *False.*   It takes 2–3 weeks to exert its effect.

(c) *False.*   Lithium is associated with hypothyroidism, due to interference with iodination.

(d) *True.*

(e) *False.*   This treatment is best reserved for the elderly age groups.

173 (a) *False.*   There is a negative feedback of ACTH production/ release from the pituitary.

(b) *True.*

(c) *True.*

(d) *True.*

(e) *True.*

174 (a) *True.*

(b) *False.*   This complication arises in pernicious anaemia if folic acid alone is administered.

(c) *True.*

(d) *False.*   It requires a further 3–6 months of iron therapy to replete body iron stores.

(e) *True.*

175 **For the relief of pain in advanced malignant disease:**
(a) The analgesic effect of NSAIDs (like aspirin) is often inadequate.
(b) Narcotic analgesics will only produce adequate analgesia if given by injection.
(c) Prochlorperazine is useful adjunctive therapy because it controls the nausea and vomiting induced by the opiate analgesics.
(d) Morphine or more potent agents of the same type are usually necessary to control the pain due to bone metastases.
(e) Constipation is often a troublesome side-effect of opiate usage.

176 **The abrupt withdrawal of the following drug(s) causes recognized adverse effects:**
(a) Phenobarbitone.
(b) Morphine.
(c) Warfarin.
(d) Propranolol.
(e) Ampicillin.

177 **Which of the following statement(s) is/are correct?**
(a) Penicillamine is the drug of first choice in rheumatoid arthritis.
(b) Aspirin will *not* prevent the progress of arthritic disease.
(c) Prednisolone will prevent the progress of arthritic disease.
(d) Codeine has useful anti-inflammatory actions.
(e) Paracetamol in clinical doses inhibits prostaglandin (PG) synthesis.

178 **Synthetic steroids like prednisolone:**
(a) Have useful central analgesic effects in the treatment of rheumatoid arthritis.
(b) Are anti-inflammatory.
(c) Cause diuresis.
(d) Can cause regression of pathologically enlarged lymph nodes.
(e) Are useful in the treatment of severe chronic asthma.

175 (a) *True.* Although the local anti-inflammatory effect of an NSAID may be useful adjunctive therapy in the treatment of bony metastases.

(b) *False.* Although the morphine-like analgesics are subject to extensive and variable first-pass metabolism, they will produce effective analgesia when administered orally.

(c) *True.* The combination of prochlorperazine with morphine or diamorphine is frequently employed.

(d) *True.* For the analgesic activity. Useful additional analgesic effects can be obtained with the concurrent use of non-steroidal anti-inflammatory drugs.

(e) *True.*

176 (a) *True.* Epilepsy may be precipitated.

(b) *True.* An acute withdrawal syndrome may be precipitated.

(c) *False.*

(d) *True.* Increased sensitivity of the beta-receptors has been shown and clinically a worsening of angina may occur.

(e) *False.*

177 (a) *False.* NSAIDs, especially salicylates, are the drugs of first choice. Penicillamine has a high incidence of adverse effects (nephrotoxicity, bone marrow depression and skin rash) and so is reserved for resistant cases.

(b) *True.*

(c) *False.*

(d) *False.*

(e) *False.*

178 (a) *False.* Steroids have no analgesic activity. Pain may be indirectly relieved as a result of their powerful anti-inflammatory effect which is sometimes useful in the treatment of severe rheumatoid disease.

(b) *True.* Anti-inflammatory activity and glucocorticoid activities are interrelated.

(c) *False.* They tend to cause fluid retention.

(d) *True.* It may therefore be useful in the management of leukaemia and lymphoma.

(e) *True.* If possible, in order to minimize the systemic adverse effects, they are best administered topically by inhaler.

179 The combined-hormone oral contraceptives:
  (a) Inhibit follicular development.
  (b) May increase hyperglycaemia.
  (c) Inhibit penetration of sperm into the uterus.
  (d) Make cervical mucus more viscous.
  (e) Produce a pseudodecidualized endometrium.

180 Which of the following statements are correct:
  (a) Renin substrate is synthesized in the liver.
  (b) Angiotensin I is converted to angiotensin II mainly in the lung.
  (c) Angiotensin I possesses 50% of the vasoconstrictor activity of angiotensin II.
  (d) Angiotensin II stimulates release of aldosterone from the adrenal cortex.
  (e) Haemorrhage increases angiotensin II production.

181 Phenytoin:
  (a) Is metabolized at higher doses according to zero-order kinetics.
  (b) Is useful in controlling the pain of diabetic neuropathy.
  (c) Is effective in psychomotor epilepsy.
  (d) Inhibits hepatic microsomal enzyme systems.
  (e) Produces sedation at anticonvulsant plasma levels.

182 In the combined-hormone oral contraceptives:
  (a) The oestrogen component causes thickening of cervical mucus.
  (b) The progestogen component inhibits ovulation.
  (c) Endogenous secretions of follicle stimulating hormone (FSH) and luteinizing hormone (LH) are increased.
  (d) The progestogen component is largely responsible for the thromboembolic side-effects.
  (e) The risk of an adverse effect is higher in women under 35 years of age.

183 Diamorphine (heroin):
  (a) Is metabolized to morphine.
  (b) Causes nausea and vomiting.
  (c) Is a respiratory depressant.
  (d) Causes pin-point pupils.
  (e) Has potent atropine-like properties.

179 (a) *True.* By inhibition of release of FSH from the pituitary.
  (b) *True.* Further impairment of carbohydrate tolerance occurs in diabetic and prediabetic women. It is not established that the 'pill' has this effect in healthy women.
  (c) *True.*⎫ This is a secondary component of the contraceptive
  (d) *True.*⎭ effect.
  (e) *True.*

180 (a) *True.*
  (b) *True.* Angiotensin converting enzyme (ACE) is located in vascular endothelial cells, particularly in the lung.
  (c) *False.* Angiotensin I is virtually inactive.
  (d) *True.* In addition to its direct vasoconstrictor effects it raises blood pressure by inducing sodium retention.
  (e) *True.* The renin–angiotensin–aldosterone system responds particularly to hypovolaemia.

181 (a) *True.* The pharmacokinetics of phenytoin are initially first order (i.e. for low plasma concentrations) but zero-order kinetics pertain at the higher plasma concentrations obtained with higher doses.
  (b) *True.* As with trigeminal neuralgia, both carbamazepine and phenytoin may be useful.
  (c) *True.*
  (d) *False.* It induces hepatic microsomal enzyme activity.
  (e) *True.*

182 (a) *True.* This is a component of the contraceptive activity.
  (b) *False.* It is the oestrogen content which suppresses.
  (c) *False.* Endogenous pituitary hormone secretion decreases and thereby inhibits ovulation.
  (d) *False.* This primarily relates to the oestrogen content.
  (e) *False.*

183 (a) *True.* It is diacetylmorphine: it is first metabolized to monoacetylmorphine and then to morphine.
  (b) *True.*
  (c) *True.*
  (d) *True.*
  (e) *False.*

184 The following drugs have the liver as their major route of elimination (for the parent drug form):
(a) Gentamicin.
(b) Propranolol.
(c) Digoxin.
(d) Frusemide.
(e) Hydralazine.

185 In the treatment of Addison's disease (primary adrenal insufficiency):
(a) Fludrocortisone may be necessary to maintain normal electrolyte balance.
(b) Steroid dosage should be increased during intercurrent illness or infection.
(c) Androgens are usually also required.
(d) Simulation of the normal circadian rhythm is conveniently achieved with twice-daily glucocorticoid administration.
(e) Dexamethasone is useful alternative therapy because of its pronounced salt-retaining effect.

186 In a woman aged 50 suffering from thyrotoxicosis:
(a) Radioiodine is the treatment of choice.
(b) If carbimazole is used, it will have to be administered for the rest of her life.
(c) Lid retraction may be helped by the administration of guanethidine eye-drops.
(d) Co-existent cardiac failure, which is often due to atrial fibrillation, is easily controlled by digoxin.
(e) Propranolol has a place in the symptomatic management.

187 When a patient has been established on a stable effective dose of the coumarin anticoagulant, warfarin:
(a) Administration of aspirin will reduce its efficacy.
(b) The introduction of phenytoin may cause haemorrhage.
(c) The majority of the circulating warfarin is bound to plasma albumin.
(d) A coagulation index of less than 5% of normal (thrombotest) is desirable.
(e) Foods containing vitamin K should be avoided.

184 (a) *False.* Exclusively glomerular filtration by the kidney.

(b) *True.* There is extensive first-pass hepatic metabolism.

(c) *False.* Only about 25% is metabolized: the remainder is eliminated by glomerular filtration.

(d) *False.* Only about 5% is metabolized: most is filtered and actively secreted by the kidney.

(e) *True.* Including hepatic acetylation.

185 (a) *True.* It has powerful mineralocorticoid activity.

(b) *True.*

(c) *False.*

(d) *True.* The physiological maintenance dose of hydrocortisone is about 30 mg daily (or prednisolone 7·5 mg daily), typically administered as 20 mg *mane* and 10 mg *nocte* (prednisolone 5 mg and 2·5 mg) to mimic the normal circadian rhythm.

(e) *False.* Dexamethasone is virtually devoid of mineralocorticoid activity.

186 (a) *True.*

(b) *False.* Approximately 50% of patients will be cured after one year's therapy.

(c) *True.*

(d) *False.* Digoxin is appropriate, but these patients have altered pharmacokinetics and pharmacodynamics for digoxin, which often achieves only a partial response despite higher than usual doses.

(e) *True.* Particularly to control symptomatic tachycardia (beta-adrenoceptor-mediated) and tremor ($beta_2$-mediated).

187 (a) *False.* The antiplatelet effects of aspirin may increase the overall anticoagulant effect.

(b) *False.* The anticoagulant effect may be reduced (i.e. the risk of thrombosis will be increased) as a result of phenytoin's induction of the hepatic enzymes which metabolize warfarin.

(c) *True.* More than 90%.

(d) *False.* The desirable range is between 5 and 15%. If less than 5% there is a significant risk of haemorrhage.

(e) *False.*

188 The following drugs can cause convulsions:
  (a) Doxapram.
  (b) Morphine.
  (c) Amitriptyline.
  (d) Digoxin.
  (e) Aminophylline.

189 The following statements about antibacterial drugs are true:
  (a) The combination of ampicillin and clavulinic acid is useful.
  (b) Tetracycline is deposited in growing bones.
  (c) Chloramphenicol is a recognized cause of aplastic anaemia.
  (d) Cephalexin is eliminated to a significant extent by active tubular secretion in the kidney.
  (e) Neomycin is the only aminoglycoside absorbed to a significant extent following oral administration.

190 The following are correct statements:
  (a) Diamorphine should be used with caution in patients suffering from chronic bronchitis.
  (b) Topical hydrocortisone is useful for localized ulcerative proctitis.
  (c) Flecainide is the treatment of choice for complete heart block.
  (d) Propranolol is useful therapy for the relief of bronchospasm.
  (e) Probenecid reduces the renal elimination of penicillin.

191 In the treatment of cancer:
  (a) Fluorouracil is effective because it inhibits purine synthesis.
  (b) Doxorubicin may cause a cardiomyopathy.
  (c) Cyclophosphamide is only effective after metabolic conversion.
  (d) Vinblastine arrests cell division in metaphase.
  (e) Bleomycin is associated with the development of pulmonary fibrosis.

188 (a) *True.*   Both doxapram and nikethamide are analeptic con-
vulsant drugs because their activating effect on the
CNS is not selective for the respiratory centre.
Doxopram retains a limited role as a respiratory
stimulant.

(b) *False.*   It is a general CNS depressant and, in the absence of the
specific anticonvulsant drug, has been used as an
emergency treatment of epilepsy. (The abrupt
withdrawal of morphine, however, from a dependent
patient may precipitate convulsions.)

(c) *True.*   Particularly in overdosage. This is in part due to the
anticholinergic effects in the CNS.

(d) *True.*   As a rare manifestion of digoxin toxicity on the CNS.

(e) *True.*   Particularly as a manifestation of toxicity.

189 (a) *True.*   This forms the proprietary preparation Augmentin,
with the clavulinic acid acting as a competitive
inhibitor of penicillinase enzymes.

(b) *True.*   Also in teeth leading to a yellow discoloration.

(c) *True.*   For this reason its use is restricted to particular
circumstances.

(d) *True.*   Both cephalosporins and penicillins are eliminated to
a significant extent by this mechanism.

(e) *False.*   Neomycin is often administered orally on the
assumption that, by not being absorbed, it will exert a
local effect within the lumen of the large intestine and
destroy intestinal organisms.

190 (a) *True.*   The opiate-induced respiratory depression is
potentially lethal as a result of their dependency on
hypoxic drive.

(b) *True.*

(c) *False.*   It may worsen heart block.

(d) *False.*   It may worsen bronchospasm by antagonism of
bronchial beta$_2$-receptors.

(e) *True.*   By interfering with its active secretion by the renal
tubules.

191 (a) *True.*   Inhibition of nuclear synthesis is the mechanism of
action of the antimetabolite drugs fluorouracil,
mercaptopurine and cytarabine.

(b) *True.*   Dose-related: leads to cardiac failure.

(c) *True.*

(d) *True.*   It interferes with messenger RNA production, as do the
other vinca alkaloids and etoposide.

(e) *True.*   Dose-related.

192 An increase in heart rate characteristically follows:
  (a) Physostigmine.
  (b) Digoxin.
  (c) Glyceryl trinitrate.
  (d) Isoprenaline.
  (e) Atenolol.

193 Which of the following drugs promote urinary loss of potassium from the body?
  (a) Spironolactone.
  (b) Amiloride.
  (c) Fludrocortisone.
  (d) Frusemide.
  (e) Carbenoxolone.

194 Which of the following may interfere with blood pressure control in a hypertensive on a regimen of a beta$_1$-blocker and a thiazide diuretic?
  (a) Salbutamol by aerosol spray.
  (b) Indomethacin.
  (c) Large doses of parenteral penicillin.
  (d) Magnesium trisilicate.
  (e) Cimetidine.

195 Which of the following drugs have hepatic enzyme-inducing properties?
  (a) Penicillin.
  (b) Diazepam.
  (c) Carbamazepine.
  (d) Isoniazid.
  (e) Cimetidine.

192 (a) *False.* This is an anticholinesterase and thus promotes cholinergic activity which leads to bradycardia.

(b) *False.* There is usually a bradycardia due to increased vagal responsiveness.

(c) *True.* Due to the reflex response to peripheral vascular dilation.

(d) *True.* As a direct result of stimulating cardiac beta$_1$-receptors and also as a reflex response to the vasodilatation from stimulating peripheral vascular beta$_2$-receptors.

(e) *False.* It is a selective beta$_1$-adrenoceptor antagonist.

193 (a) *False.* This drug acts on the distal tubule and collecting ducts to interfere with aldosterone-induced potassium loss. It acts therefore as an aldosterone antagonist.

(b) *False.* This drug prevents the loss of potassium ions from the distal tubule and collecting ducts by interfering with both aldosterone-dependent and non-aldosterone dependent mechanisms.

(c) *True.* This is a synthetic mineralocorticoid whose actions mimic aldosterone and thereby promote the urinary loss of potassium in exchange for a retention of sodium.

(d) *True.* Loop diuretics, such as frusemide and bumetanide, and also the thiazide diuretics, promote urinary loss of potassium as well as sodium.

(e) *True.* Carbenoxolone has an aldosterone-like effect in promoting potassium loss and sodium retention.

194 (a) *False.* The beta$_2$-agonist by this route will not influence blood pressure.

(b) *True.* Both beta-blocker and diuretic action may be antagonized by effects on renal prostaglandins.

(c) *True.* If the sodium salt of penicillin is given.

(d) *False.* No effect would be expected.

(e) *False.* Although cimetidine may inhibit metabolism of some beta-blockers, this will not prevent and may enhance their effects.

195 (a) *False.* Enzyme induction is not a feature of penicillins.

(b) *False.*

(c) *True.* Also with other anticonvulsants, e.g. phenytoin.

(d) *False.*

(e) *False.* This drug has enzyme-inhibiting properties.

196 The following drug side-effects are well recognized:
   (a) Constipation with atenolol.
   (b) Deafness with streptomycin.
   (c) Proteinuria with penicillamine.
   (d) Increased urinary frequency with disopyramide.
   (e) Headache with glyceryl trinitrate.

197 In paracetamol overdosage:
   (a) Deep coma typically develops within 24 hours.
   (b) N-acetylcysteine is indicated when plasma paracetamol levels are very high.
   (c) Pulmonary fibrosis is a late complication.
   (d) Previous alcoholic liver disease predisposes to severe liver damage.
   (e) Forced alkaline diuresis is indicated.

198 Carbamazepine:
   (a) Is useful in the treatment of trigeminal neuralgia.
   (b) Is useful in the treatment of thyrotoxicosis.
   (c) Is useful in the treatment of epilepsy.
   (d) Is associated with bone marrow depression.
   (e) Is associated with ataxia, drowsiness and slurred speech when plasma concentrations reach toxic levels.

199 Combined oestrogen–progestogen oral contraceptive agents:
   (a) Suppress pituitary secretion of LH and FSH.
   (b) Act primarily by altering the physical properties of cervical mucus.
   (c) Are relatively contraindicated in hypertensive women.
   (d) May precipitate migraine.
   (e) Are associated with an increased risk of thromboembolic disease.

200 Conventional antihistamines (H_1 antagonists), for example cyclizine and diphenhydramine:
   (a) Act by competitive inhibition at the cellular receptor site for histamine.
   (b) Antagonize histamine-stimulated gastric acid production.
   (c) Have useful antiemetic actions.
   (d) Are useful in bronchial asthma.
   (e) Are the drugs of choice for the immediate emergency treatment of anaphylactic shock.

196 (a) *False.*   Diarrhoea is a more usual complication.

   (b) *True.*   The aminoglycoside group damage the eighth cranial nerve as a toxic effect.

   (c) *True.*

   (d) *False.*   The anticholinergic properties of disopyramide cause urinary retention.

   (e) *True.*   Due to dilatation of intracranial blood vessels.

197 (a) *False.*   Coma is rarely a feature of paracetamol overdose.

   (b) *True.*   It prevents the formation of paracetamol's toxic metabolites which cause liver (and kidney) damage.

   (c) *False.*

   (d) *True.*   Probably by increasing enzyme activity and thereby promoting the formation of toxic metabolites.

   (e) *False.*   This technique is useful for enhancing renal elimination of drug: aspirin and phenobarbitone are the commonest examples.

198 (a) *True.*   May also be useful in post-herpetic and diabetic neuralgia.

   (b) *False.*   The relevant drug is carbimazole.

   (c) *True.*   Both for grand mal and petit mal.

   (d) *True.*   A rare side-effect is agranulocytosis.

   (e) *True.*   True, although the therapeutic range is less well defined than for other drugs, because of its active metabolite, carbamazepine-10, 11-epoxide.

199 (a) *True.*

   (b) *False.*   This is a secondary effect.

   (c) *True.*

   (d) *True.*

   (e) *True.*

200 (a) *True.*

   (b) *False.*   Gastric acid secretion is dependent upon the H_2-receptor.

   (c) *True.*

   (d) *False.*

   (e) *False.*   Adrenaline is the drug of choice for the emergency treatment. The antihistamines may usefully prevent further histamine release.

SECTION III

201.1 **A man aged 38 years, who smokes 20 cigarettes daily, is noted at an insurance medical examination to have a blood pressure of 204/118 mmHg. Two weeks later his general practitioner confirms that his blood pressure is elevated at 198/114 (the average of two readings, following 10 minutes recumbency):**
  (a) The patient should be reassured, given no treatment and reviewed four weeks later.
  (b) The patient has an increased risk of cerebrovascular accident.
  (c) The patient requires a full clinical examination, including ophthalmoscopy of the retina.
  (d) There is good evidence that he should benefit from antihypertensive therapy.
  (e) The patient should be strongly advised to stop smoking.

201.2 **When it is decided to start antihypertensive medication in this patient, the preferred treatment for initial therapy is likely to be:**
  (a) Single-drug therapy with a beta-blocker.
  (b) Dietary salt restriction (20 mEq Na daily).
  (c) Hydralazine monotherapy.
  (d) A thiazide diuretic.
  (e) Combination therapy with atenolol, frusemide and prazosin.

201.3 **Further enquiry elicits that the patient has past history of intermittent seasonal asthma and further investigations reveal that he has evidence of ischaemic heart disease (ST segment elevation) on exercise electrocardiography. If it is decided to treat him with a beta-blocker:**
  (a) A cardioselective beta-blocker would be preferable to a non-selective beta-blocker.
  (b) Propranolol would be preferable to atenolol.
  (c) Beta-blocker therapy is sometimes associated with the development of hallucinations and nightmares.
  (d) Tachyarrhythmias and angina pectoris are possible side-effects of beta-blockers.
  (e) Symptoms of intermittent claudication are likely to be improved by beta-blockers.

201.4 **In view of his previous history of asthma it is decided that a calcium antagonist drug is more appropriate:**
  (a) Verapamil is a reasonable choice.
  (b) Ankle oedema is a well-recognized side-effect of nifedipine.
  (c) Verapamil and atenolol is an established, safe and effective combination for hypertension complicated by ischaemic heart disease.
  (d) Nifedipine is an alternative to verapamil in this patient.
  (e) Headache may be precipitated by nifedipine.

201.1 (a) *False.*   **201.2** (a) *True.*   **201.3** (a) *True.*   **201.4** (a) *True.*
     (b) *True.*   (b) *False.*   (b) *False.*   (b) *True.*
     (c) *True.*   (c) *False.*   (c) *True.*   (c) *False.*
     (d) *True.*   (d) *False.*   (d) *False.*   (d) *True.*
     (e) *True.*   (e) *False.*   (e) *False.*   (e) *True.*

The diagnosis of hypertension should not be based on an isolated reading. Typically, two readings, obtained under restful conditions, on separate occasions, are sufficient. There is established epidemiological evidence that this patient's level of blood pressure is associated with an increased risk of cardiac failure, cerebral vascular accident, renal failure and possibly myocardial infarction. These risks can be improved by satisfactory blood pressure control and additionally by the correction of associated risk factors, of which the most important is cigarette smoking. A routine clinical examination is mandatory initially in order to exclude the occasional secondary type of hypertension and additionally to assess any clinical evidence of target organ damage such as cardiomegaly or hypertensive retinopathy. As yet there is no 'ideal' antihypertensive drug. A beta-adrenoceptor antagonist, especially in the younger middle-age group, is currently the drug of first choice. Dietary salt restriction to very low levels is unpalatable for most patients and has not been shown to be of long-term benefit.

Treatment with drugs such as hydralazine and prazosin, which have vasodilator actions, is optimally undertaken in combination regimens with a beta-blocker and/or a diuretic, in order to overcome the reflex mechanisms induced by peripheral vasodilatation. The great majority of patients will be successfully controlled on therapy with one or two drugs and only about 10% will require more complex regimens. The cardioselective beta-blockers are generally considered to be preferable in the treatment of hypertension because the side-effects attributable to blockade of $beta_2$-receptors, including bronchospasm and peripheral vasoconstriction, are less likely to occur. Accordingly, beta-blockers are relatively contraindicated in patients with bronchial asthma and peripheral vascular disease, but they may be relatively positively indicated in patients with angina pectoris and a tendency to cardiac tachyarrythmias. Side-effects from beta-blockers also include CNS effects, but these appear to be associated most frequently with the lipid-soluble beta-blockers, particularly propranolol, and may give rise to hallucinations and vivid nightmares. Because of concerns about the long-term adverse effects of thiazide diuretics particularly, but also because beta-blockers are not free of side-effects, there has been a recent trend towards the use of other drugs which appear to be relatively free of side-effects, although their long-term efficacy and safety remain to be established. This is particularly true of the calcium antagonists and the angiotensin converting enzyme inhibitors which have recently been introduced.

A 62-year-old retired miner with a long history of chronic obstructive airways disease is admitted to the chest clinic with severe dyspnoea and an elevated temperature. The diagnosis of an acute exacerbation of chronic bronchitis is made.

202.1 The following are appropriate steps in his management:
(a) Delay in starting antibiotic treatment until the result of sputum culture is known.
(b) A 'broad-spectrum' antibiotic.
(c) Intravenous benzylpenicillin.
(d) High-concentration oxygen therapy.
(e) Salbutamol by nebulizer.

202.2 The patient is started on ampicillin and salbutamol and within 24 hours of admission the pyrexia settles but severe dyspnoea persists:
(a) Antibiotic therapy should be stopped.
(b) The initial diagnosis should be reviewed.
(c) Salbutamol should be given as an oral therapy which is more effective.
(d) Additional therapy with theophylline may be indicated.
(e) Additional therapy with high-dosage prednisolone may be indicated.

202.3 Sputum culture grows coliform organisms and the blood gas analysis shows a low Po_2 and an elevated Pco_2. The chest X-ray shows signs of infection and pulmonary venous congestion.
(a) Ampicillin is active against most coliform organisms.
(b) Co-trimoxazole is an alternative 'broad-spectrum' antibacterial.
(c) Chest physiotherapy is definitely contraindicated because of the low Po_2.
(d) High-concentration oxygen therapy must be continued because of the low Po_2.
(e) Frusemide is indicated.

202.4 The patient's general condition improves over the next few days, but he develops a maculopapular rash and diarrhoea:
(a) A skin rash is a common side-effect of ampicillin.
(b) Agranulocytosis is a common side-effect of ampicillin.
(c) He is obviously 'allergic' to penicillin which he should be told to avoid in future.
(d) Diarrhoea is a common side-effect of ampicillin.
(e) Secondary fungal infection of the throat is a complication of 'broad-spectrum' antibiotics.

202.1 (a) *False.*   **202.2** (a) *False.*   **202.3** (a) *True.*   **202.4** (a) *True.*
    (b) *True.*   (b) *False.*   (b) *True.*   (b) *False.*
    (c) *False.*   (c) *False.*   (c) *False.*   (c) *False.*
    (d) *False.*   (d) *True.*   (d) *False.*   (d) *True.*
    (e) *True.*   (e) *True.*   (e) *True.*   (e) *True.*

Exacerbations of chronic obstructive airways disease are frequently precipitated by intercurrent infections. Antibacterial treatment should be initiated as quickly as possible on a 'best guess' basis, and for this purpose broad-spectrum antibiotics, such as ampicillin or co-trimoxazole or a cephalosporin, are suitable. A more specific choice of antibiotic would only be indicated if there were particular reasons for suspecting an organism such as legionnella (erythromycin or rifampicin) or pneumococcus (benzylpenicillin). In addition to the antibiotic it is usually necessary to use bronchodilator therapy such as the beta$_2$ agonist salbutamol and/or the direct bronchodilator theophylline. Salbutamol is best administered by a nebulizer or by inhaler in order to deliver the drug directly to the bronchial tree. If it is administered by mouth then the systemic side-effects are usually troublesome, particularly a feeling of nervousness and tremulousness. Antibiotic therapy is best continued for about five days, but evidence of bronchoconstriction may persist even after the initial infection appears to have been controlled. If the response to salbutamol plus theophylline is inadequate then additional therapy with corticosteroids may be necessary. Corticosteroids in this circumstance 'sensitize' the bronchi to respond to the other drugs. Additional therapies which may be indicated are diuretics, if there is evidence of pulmonary congestion or complicating cardiac heart failure; oxygen therapy which should be controlled, typically at 24 or 28%, because of the risks of further respiratory depression and CO_2 narcosis (the patient with COAD is dependent upon hypoxic drive); and chest physiotherapy to relieve obstruction due to retained secretions. A low Po_2 is not a contraindication to physiotherapy.

    Ampicillin is one of the antibiotics most frequently used in this circumstance because of its broad spectrum of activity, which includes coliform organisms, and because of its relative safety and freedom from serious side-effects. Nevertheless, ampicillin frequently causes minor side-effects, including a maculopapular skin rash in about 10% of patients and diarrhoea in a similar percentage. The skin rash attributable to ampicillin is rarely a genuine penicillin allergy and there is no need for the patient subsequently to avoid other types of penicillin for this reason alone. A sore throat is a relatively common complication of broad-spectrum antibiotic therapy, particularly if this is prolonged, and typically indicates a secondary infection of the throat with fungal organisms. It is not an indication of an underlying more serious abnormality of white cells.

203.1 A 57-year-old accountant is admitted to hospital complaining of severe breathlessness and crushing central chest pain of two hours' duration. The house physician finds that the patient has a rapid pulse rate and signs of pulmonary oedema and before contacting his registrar makes the following treatment decisions:

(a) Morphine should not be given to relieve the pain as it may worsen breathlessness by depressing the respiratory centre.

(b) Intravenous frusemide should be given to treat the pulmonary oedema.

(c) Controlled (24%) oxygen therapy is best for this type of breathlessness.

(d) The patient should lie flat and rest as quietly as possible.

(e) Propranolol should be given immediately to slow the rapid heart rate.

203.2 The rapid pulse is found to be due to atrial fibrillation with a ventricular rate of 170/min. The following are appropriate immediate treatments for the atrial fibrillation:

(a) Cardioversion with DC shock.

(b) Intravenous lignocaine.

(c) Intravenous verapamil.

(d) Intravenous aminophylline.

(e) Oral isosorbide dinitrate.

203.3 The registrar, however, prefers digoxin. He explains:

(a) Intravenous digoxin will satisfactorily control the heart rate within five minutes.

(b) Digoxin acts on the AV conduction system to diminish the number of atrial impulses reaching the ventricles.

(c) Digoxin inhibits the vagus and thus slows the heart rate.

(d) Reversion to sinus rhythm is the expected consequence of digoxin therapy.

(e) Potassium depletion protects against digoxin toxicity.

203.4 The patient is continued on oral digoxin and frusemide. On reviewing the patient the next day the consultant finds that he has severe renal impairment and makes the following observations:

(a) The patient's maintenance dose of digoxin should be reduced because he has severe renal impairment.

(b) Bendrofluazide is indicated in place of frusemide.

(c) Morphine should have been used as it improves pulmonary oedema by reducing venous return to the lungs.

(d) A potential side-effect of long-term digoxin therapy is gynaecomastia.

(e) A potential side-effect of long-term diuretic therapy is impairment of glucose tolerance.

203.1 (a) *False.*   **203.2** (a) *True.*   **203.3** (a) *False.*   **203.4** (a) *True.*
    (b) *True.*   (b) *False.*   (b) *True.*   (b) *False.*
    (c) *False.*   (c) *True.*   (c) *False.*   (c) *True.*
    (d) *False.*   (d) *False.*   (d) *False.*   (d) *True.*
    (e) *False.*   (e) *False.*   (e) *False.*   (e) *True.*

Acute pulmonary oedema is a frequent complication of acute myocardial infarction whether or not atrial fibrillation also develops. The patient should rest in an upright position, as even the mild gravitational effect of lying flat often worsens the pulmonary congestion. Morphine should be given both to relieve the subjective component of dyspnoea and distress and also because it reduces 'pre-load' and thereby tends to relieve the pulmonary oedema. While both intravenous aminophylline and isosorbide dinitrate may be useful in the treatment of pulmonary oedema they do not have any specific effect in atrial fibrillation. Aminophylline acts to relieve bronchial constriction and also to promote renal vasodilatation and diuresis. Isosorbide dinitrate acts as a venodilator and thus as a pre-load-reducing agent. In acute pulmonary oedema neither morphine nor high-dose oxygen therapy, which should also be administered, should be withheld for fear of depressing the respiratory centre unless there is very convincing evidence of chronic obstructive airways disease. Intravenous diuretic therapy is particularly useful in promoting fluid removal and also has a mild venodilator effect. Atrial fibrillation in this circumstance is best controlled with digoxin. Conventional antiarrhythmic therapy, such as lignocaine or disopyramide, is not usually effective and has the further disadvantage of depressant effects on cardiac function. Cardioversion with DC shock is a possible alternative to try to convert the rhythm back to sinus rhythm. The digoxin may be administered intravenously, and while some reduction in the heart rate may occur within 5 or 10 minutes, full control of the ventricular rate is not usually achieved until further doses have been given over a period of hours. Digoxin occasionally causes a reversion to sinus rhythm, but its major beneficial effect in atrial fibrillation is to diminish the number of atrial impulses which reach the ventricles by depressing AV conduction. It has a mild effect on the vagus nerve, which it stimulates, and thereby tends to slow the heart rate. Potassium depletion sensitizes the heart to the effects of digoxin and this is obviously a potential problem if diuretic therapy is also administered. Digoxin accumulation occurs, with its risk of toxicity, if there is renal impairment, and the dosage may require to be reduced in this circumstance. If the renal impairment is severe then loop diuretics such as frusemide are likely to be necessary, as thiazide diuretics will be relatively ineffective. Digoxin is not free of long-term side-effects, and because of its steroid structure gynaecomastia is a recognized complication in men. The long-term effects of diuretic therapy include disturbance of carbohydrate metabolism and urate retention, but frank diabetes mellitus and gout are rare.

204.1 A 45-year-old woman with a 15-year history of asthma is maintained on oral theophylline therapy (450 mg twice daily). Despite taking double her normal dose of theophylline for the past two days she becomes increasingly breathless and wheezy. She is seen by the casualty officer who correctly offers as first-choice therapy for the relief of bronchospasm and general distress:
(a) Diazepam.
(b) Hydrocortisone.
(c) Propranolol.
(d) Salbutamol.
(e) Morphine.

204.2 The casualty officer then decides that aminophylline is appropriate therapy:
(a) A rapid (30 seconds) intravenous bolus injection is the correct mode of administration.
(b) There is a significant risk of producing theophylline toxicity with this therapy in this patient.
(c) Theophylline toxicity may manifest as convulsions.
(d) Aminophylline would have been contraindicated if the patient had already received salbutamol.
(e) As well as its bronchodilator activity, aminophylline is a weak central respiratory stimulant.

204.3 The following are true of the theophylline group of bronchodilators:
(a) They act as selective beta$_2$ agonists and thereby induce bronchodilatation.
(b) Tachycardia and cardiac dysrhythmias are recognized side-effects.
(c) They are extensively metabolized in the liver.
(d) The dosage should be decreased in even mild degrees of renal failure to avoid toxic accumulation of the drug.
(e) The maintenance dosage schedule can be calculated from the peak blood concentration following a single intravenous dose of aminophylline.

204.4 This patient makes an uneventful recovery following treatment with theophylline and salbutamol. If she had failed to respond, the following additional treatments would have been of likely benefit:
(a) A short course of prednisolone.
(b) Sodium cromoglycate by inhalation.
(c) Hydralazine.
(d) Ipratropium bromide by inhalation.
(e) Beclomethasone dipropionate by inhalation.

204.1 (a) *False.*   **204.2** (a) *False.*   **204.3** (a) *False.*   **204.4** (a) *True.*
      (b) *True.*   (b) *True.*   (b) *True.*   (b) *False.*
      (c) *False.*   (c) *True.*   (c) *True.*   (c) *False.*
      (d) *True.*   (d) *False.*   (d) *False.*   (d) *True.*
      (e) *False.*   (e) *True.*   (e) *False.*   (e) *True.*

Asthma is a disease of reversible airways obstruction and accordingly should be first treated with bronchodilator therapies such as the beta$_2$ agonists salbutamol or terbutaline; the direct bronchodilator theophylline derivatives; or the anticholinergic agents such as ipratropium. Acutely the theophylline derivative of choice is aminophylline by intravenous administration. Care is required with a slow intravenous injection, typically over 5–10 minutes, as rapid bolus administration may result in a direct cardiotoxic effect with ventricular arrythmias. An additional complication of intravenous therapy is the risk of producing toxic plasma levels if the patient has already been receiving oral theophylline treatment in the preceding few days. High plasma levels of theophylline are associated with convulsions in addition to tachycardia and cardiac dysrhythmias. Other bronchodilator therapies, with either beta agonists or anticholinergics, are not contraindications to intravenous aminophylline. Aminophylline, which exerts its effect by a 'direct' action, also has additional effects as a weak vasodilator, particularly of the renal arteries, and it also has a central respiratory stimulant effect. It is extensively metabolized by the liver, and dosage adjustments may be required if there is functional liver impairment. Mild degrees of renal impairment do not significantly affect theophylline kinetics. Because of the risks of toxicity and the establishment of a therapeutic range, theophylline dosage can be controlled by measuring the plasma drug levels. However a single peak drug level is not adequate for this purpose. In the treatment of acute bronchial asthma, although CO_2 retention is not a chronic problem, it is best to avoid drugs which are potential respiratory depressants. Propranolol is, of course, contraindicated because its antagonism of bronchial beta$_2$-receptors may exacerbate the tendency to bronchial constriction. Corticosteroid therapy is often useful in severe asthma and can be administered intravenously, orally, or by inhalation. Apart from reducing oedema and inflammation of the bronchial mucosa, corticosteroids seem to exert a sensitizing effect to render the bronchial trees more responsive to the effects of other bronchodilator therapies. Sodium cromoglycate is not useful in the relief of bronchospasm but has a place in the management and prophylaxis of young patients in whom there is a significant allergic component underlying their tendency to asthma. Conversely, ipratropium by inhalation is often useful adjunctive therapy in the asthma of older patients. Systemic therapy with anticholinergic drugs is unhelpful because the systemic side-effects are unacceptable. Hydralazine is inappropriate therapy because it has no bronchodilator activity although it is a direct-acting vasodilator suitable for the treatment of hypertension.

205.1 A general practitioner is called to see a 42-year-old man with severe central chest pain. He diagnoses acute myocardial infarction and notes a rapid pulse with frequent irregularities of rhythm. Before referring the patient to hospital he considers giving an antiarrhythmic drug:
(a) Intravenous digoxin is appropriate for atrial fibrillation.
(b) Oral mexiletine would be useful for ventricular ectopic beats.
(c) Intramuscular atropine will be useful.
(d) Intramuscular lignocaine relieves cardiac pain by means of its local anaesthetic activity.
(e) Intravenous metoprolol may precipitate pulmonary oedema.

205.2 On arrival at the coronary care unit the patient is noted to have frequent multifocal ventricular ectopic beats:
(a) An intravenous bolus of lignocaine is appropriate therapy.
(b) Renal function is an important determinant in deciding the rate of intravenous lignocaine infusion.
(c) Low-dose lignocaine infusion is of proven value in prophylaxis against primary ventricular fibrillation.
(d) Lignocaine acts through beta-adrenergic receptor blockade.
(e) An advantage of lignocaine is that it does not cause severe hypotension.

205.3 Satisfactory control of ventricular ectopic activity is achieved but unifocal supraventricular beats occur frequently and there are short runs of supraventricular tachycardia:
(a) This is a dangerous dysrhythmia and treatment is mandatory.
(b) A beta-adrenergic blocking agent is likely to be helpful.
(c) Intravenous verapamil is contraindicated if a beta-adrenergic blocking drug has already been given.
(d) Disopyramide may control both ventricular and supraventricular ectopic rhythms.
(e) DC shock is urgently indicated.

205.4 The patient progresses satisfactorily but withdrawal of parenteral antidysrhythmic therapy is associated with a return of ectopic activity:
(a) It would be reasonable to continue disopyramide orally.
(b) Antidysrhythmic activity of disopyramide is related to plasma concentration.
(c) Disopyramide is solely eliminated by the liver, so that hepatic congestion will greatly influence the dose given.
(d) Urinary retention and dry mouth are recognized side-effects of disopyramide.
(e) Disopyramide will provide adequate protection given once daily to patients with normal renal function.

205.1 (a) *False.*   **205.2** (a) *True.*   **205.3** (a) *False.*   **205.4** (a) *True.*
        (b) *True.*   (b) *False.*   (b) *True.*   (b) *True.*
        (c) *False.*   (c) *False.*   (c) *True.*   (c) *False.*
        (d) *False.*   (d) *False.*   (d) *True.*   (d) *True.*
        (e) *True.*   (e) *True.*   (e) *False.*   (e) *False.*

In the treatment of the arrhythmias complicating acute myocardial infarction the class I antiarrhythmic agents are generally preferred for depressing ventricular ectopic rhythms. Mexiletine (class Ib) may be administered both orally and intravenously and is therefore useful for suppressing ventricular ectopic beats and other ventricular arrythmias. Because of its extensive first-pass metabolism lignocaine requires to be administered intravenously, and therapy is typically initiated with an intravenous bolus injection followed by an intravenous infusion. Lignocaine is also a class I antiarrhythmic agent (it has no effect on beta-adrenoceptors) and it is relatively free of side-effects, although toxic levels are associated with central nervous system disturbance. Disopyramide is a class Ib antiarrythmic which has activity against both supraventricular and ventricular arrythmias. It can be administered both orally and intravenously, and as its elimination is dependent upon both renal and hepatic function care must be taken if there is hepatic or renal impairment. Measurement of plasma drug levels is useful in controlling the drug regimen to obtain therapeutically effective plasma concentrations, but side-effects of an anticholinergic type, including urinary retention, dry mouth and visual disturbance, are recognized even at normal levels. If administered orally disopyramide requires administration two or three times each day. Supraventricular rhythm disturbances are less serious in the setting of acute myocardial infarction, and only if there is an associated haemodynamic upset would DC shock be urgently indicated. Other therapies provide a means of controlling supraventricular arrythmias, including beta-adrenoceptor antagonists such as metoprolol, although this has the potential disadvantage of precipitating left ventricular failure; intravenous verapamil, although this may produce profound negative effects on cardiac conduction and cardiac contractility, particularly if a beta-blocker has been previously administered; digoxin, although this is best reserved for the treatment of atrial fibrillation and atropine if there is a tendency to bradyarrythmias.

206.1 A 58-year-old housewife presents herself to the casualty department with a two-hour history of excruciating severe pain arising from the left loin, radiating to the groin, and associated with symptoms of dysuria and haematuria. The casualty officer suspects ureteric colic and makes the following recommendations:
   (a) A non-steroidal anti-inflammatory drug (such as indomethacin) is indicated.
   (b) Analgesics should be withheld until the diagnosis is confirmed.
   (c) Intramuscular pethidine is contraindicated.
   (d) Morphine should not be given because of the risk of addiction.
   (e) Analgesia is best combined with an antispasmodic such as propantheline.

206.2 He decides that intravenous morphine should be given. The following adverse effects might be observed:
   (a) Nausea and vomiting.
   (b) Diarrhoea.
   (c) An increase in blood pressure as a result of peripheral vasoconstriction.
   (d) Miosis.
   (e) Difficulty with micturition.

206.3 Unfortunately, about 15 minutes after the injection, the patient develops cyanosis and hypoventilation:
   (a) Respiratory depression is due to a direct effect of morphine on opioid receptors in the brain stem.
   (b) Opiates cause pooling of venous blood in the lungs, resulting in reduced lung compliance.
   (c) Intravenous nikethamide should be given immediately.
   (d) Intravenous naloxone will reverse the respiratory depression without antagonizing the analgesic effect.
   (e) Assisted ventilation may be required.

206.4 Morphine-like drugs achieve their effects:
   (a) Only after intravenous administration.
   (b) Optimally, when the serum concentration is maintained within a narrow therapeutic range.
   (c) By interfering with bradykinin synthesis.
   (d) By acting on specific opioid receptors in the central nervous system.
   (e) By inhibiting prostaglandin synthetase activity.

206.1 (a) *False.*   **206.2** (a) *True.*   **206.3** (a) *True.*   **206.4** (a) *False.*
       (b) *False.*   (b) *False.*   (b) *False.*   (b) *False.*
       (c) *False.*   (c) *False.*   (c) *False.*   (c) *False.*
       (d) *False.*   (d) *True.*   (d) *False.*   (d) *True.*
       (e) *True.*   (e) *False.*   (e) *True.*   (e) *False.*

Renal or ureteric colic is extremely painful and if this clinical diagnosis is made there is no reason for withholding analgesic therapy simply in order to confirm the diagnosis with X-rays (which are often negative). Simple analgesics and non-steroidal anti-inflammatory drugs are inadequate for this pain, and opioid analgesics are usually required. Theoretically, pethidine, which does not promote spasm of smooth muscle, is the drug of choice, but both pethidine and morphine may be safely and effectively administered in combination with an antispasmodic agent such as propantheline. There is no concern about opiate addiction with respect to this acute condition, but intravenous morphine has other adverse effects which typically include nausea and vomiting. Small unreactive pupils are a classical effect of opiates, and a tendency to constipation is also a common occurrence. Blood pressure tends to fall as a result of peripheral venodilatation but there are no difficulties with micturition. The major immediate complication of morphine administration is respiratory depression as a consequence of a direct effect on opiate receptors in the brain stem. This effect can be reversed by the selective opiate antagonist drug naloxone. There is not yet a therapeutic agent which can selectively act on the opiate receptors which modulate pain without also affecting the receptors for respiration. Thus, reversal of respiratory depression is accompanied by loss of analgesic effect. The respiratory stimulant drug nikethamide should now be avoided in this and other circumstances, because its potential disadvantages, particularly seizures, outweigh its benefits. Naloxone is safer and more effective. Occasionally, assisted ventilation may be required if treatment with naloxone proves inadequate. Morphine and its derivatives are effective both orally and intravenously and there is no simple relationship between serum concentrations and the drug effect. They act by stimulating specific receptors in the central nervous system and they have no significant effect on prostaglandin synthetase activity which is an effect of the non-steroidal anti-inflammatory group of drugs.

A known epileptic, a 19-year-old apprentice mechanic, is admitted to the casualty department in status epilepticus.

207.1 The following drug regimens are appropriate as initial treatments:
(a) Diazepam intravenously.
(b) Phenytoin intramuscularly.
(c) Phenobarbitone in a large oral dose.
(d) Chlormethiazole by intravenous infusion.
(e) Intravenous thiopentone and mechanical ventilation.

207.2 The patient's routine anticonvulsant therapy is reported to be phenytoin:
(a) This should be stopped at once:
(b) Phenytoin acts by inhibiting gamma-aminobutyric acid (GABA).
(c) As well as being anticonvulsant, phenytoin has anti-arrhythmic properties.
(d) Phenytoin can only be given orally.
(e) Phenytoin demonstrates dose-dependent pharmacokinetics.

207.3 On measurement of the phenytoin plasma concentration, the drug is found to be within the therapeutic range. Additional anticonvulsant therapy is considered. The following statements about other types of anticonvulsant therapy are true:
(a) Phenytoin and phenobarbitone act synergistically.
(b) The kinetics of sodium valproate are altered by enzyme induction caused by phenytoin.
(c) Phenobarbitone often causes jaundice.
(d) Phenobarbitone is the drug of choice in this young age group.
(e) Carbamazepine is mainly eliminated by the kidney and should be used with care in renal insufficiency.

207.4 It is decided to change his treatment to carbamazepine. The following are well-recognized side-effects of long-term treatment with carbamazepine:
(a) Gum hypertrophy.
(b) Osteomalacia.
(c) Leucopenia.
(d) Diplopia.
(e) Skin rash.

207.1 (a) *True.*   **207.2** (a) *False.*   **207.3** (a) *False.*   **207.4** (a) *False.*
    (b) *False.*   (b) *False.*   (b) *True.*   (b) *False.*
    (c) *False.*   (c) *True.*   (c) *False.*   (c) *True.*
    (d) *True.*   (d) *False.*   (d) *False.*   (d) *True.*
    (e) *False.*   (e) *False.*   (e) *False.*   (e) *True.*

Status epilepticus is a medical emergency for which bolus doses of intravenous diazepam (or clonazepam) are often successfully employed. An infusion of chlormethiazole or an intravenous injection of phenytoin or phenobarbitone are also appropriate therapies. Obviously drug administration by the oral route is virtually impossible in this circumstance, and the intramuscular administration of phenytoin is inappropriate because the drug is very poorly and irregularly absorbed from depot injection sites. While intravenous thiopentone and assisted ventilation may be necessary in severe cases, where some of the above therapies have failed, it is not appropriate as an initial management step. Phenobarbitone has long been established as an anticonvulsant agent, but sodium valproate, carbamazepine and phenytoin have now superseded it in rank order of preference in young people, particularly with regard to side-effects. Phenobarbitone has the additional established drawback that withdrawal of long-term therapy is often associated with 'rebound' occurrence of seizures. This is not clearly established for other anticonvulsant therapies but, on empirical grounds, abrupt therapeutic changes are not recommended. Phenobarbitone and phenytoin share a tendency to cause gum hypertrophy, osteomalacia and hirsutism during long-term therapy, but there is no evidence of bone marrow depression. However, leucopenia and thrombocytopenia have been associated with carbamazepine, and skin rash occurs in about 3%. Because of their enzyme-inducing properties, both phenytoin and phenobarbitone (and to a lesser extent carbamazepine) may alter the pharmacokinetics of other drugs which are eliminated via the liver, including sodium valproate. This enzyme-inducing capacity of phenobarbitone has been utilized in the treatment of jaundice in neonates whose enzyme capacity is underdeveloped. Both sodium valproate, which acts by promoting the synthesis of the inhibitory neurotransmitter gamma-aminobutyric acid, and carbamazepine are now preferred anticonvulsants for children. The precise mechanism of action of phenobarbitone, phenytoin and carbamazepine remains unknown, and while their effects, to some extent, are additive they are not synergistic.

A 49-year-old businesswoman is referred to the out-patient clinic with the complaint of pain, swelling and stiffness of both hands for six months. On examination she has features of active rheumatoid arthritis.

208.1 The following treatments should be considered as first line:
(a) Dihydrocodeine.
(b) Salicylates in low doses (2 g/day).
(c) Piroxicam.
(d) Prednisolone.
(e) Ibuprofen.

208.2 She is commenced on treatment with indomethacin:
(a) Indomethacin acts by inhibiting prostaglandin synthesis.
(b) It has a tendency to cause fluid retention, particularly in the elderly.
(c) It is a much stronger anti-inflammatory agent than aspirin.
(d) It causes much less gastrointestinal disturbance than aspirin.
(e) It has a tendency to cause headache.

208.3 Over the next five years, despite treatment with various non-steroidal anti-inflammatory agents, this patient's rheumatoid disease remains active and she is started on prednisolone:
(a) Prednisolone similarly acts by inhibiting prostaglandin synthetase activity.
(b) It diminishes the inflammatory response, in part, by its effect on white cells.
(c) The anti-inflammatory effects of prednisolone are additional to those of indomethacin.
(d) Prednisone is metabolized in the liver to prednisolone, which is the active form.
(e) Betamethasone, because of its very powerful anti-inflammatory effect, is preferable to prednisolone in rheumatoid arthritis.

208.4 Prednisolone is relatively contraindicated if the following conditions are present:
(a) Peptic ulcer.
(b) Thrombocytopenia.
(c) Hypertension.
(d) Exfoliative dermatitis.
(e) Congestive cardiac failure.

208.1 (a) *False.*   **208.2** (a) *True.*   **208.3** (a) *False.*   **208.4** (a) *True.*
   (b) *False.*   (b) *True.*   (b) *True.*   (b) *False.*
   (c) *True.*   (c) *True.*   (c) *True.*   (c) *True.*
   (d) *False.*   (d) *False.*   (d) *True.*   (d) *False.*
   (e) *True.*   (e) *True.*   (e) *False.*   (e) *True.*

The initial management of active rheumatoid arthritis should include a non-steroidal anti-inflammatory drug, such as indomethacin or ibuprofen. Aspirin (salicylates) which is the standard anti-inflammatory drug requires to be administered in high dosage, typically in excess of 2 g daily, in order to achieve a major anti-inflammatory effect. At this stage in treatment specific antirheumatoid agents such as gold or penicillamine are not indicated, and similarly corticosteroids should be withheld until a later stage. All of these drugs have serious potential adverse effects. Simple analgesic and opiate derivatives are inappropriate for the routine treatment of rheumatoid disease. Indomethacin, which is a powerful anti-inflammatory drug, acts by inhibiting the synthesis of prostaglandins. This is the mechanism common to all anti-inflammatory agents, but it remains unclear whether or not this is their sole anti-inflammatory mechanism. For comparable anti-inflammatory actions there is no evidence that indomethacin causes significantly less gastrointestinal disturbance than aspirin, and in addition indomethacin causes a number of other side-effects, including fluid retention, particularly in the elderly, and a troublesome muzzy headache which is dose-related. If prednisolone therapy is required it may usefully be combined in anti-inflammatory terms with a non-steroidal anti-inflammatory drug. There is some risk, however, of an additive effect in causing gastrointestinal side-effects. The precise mechanism of action of prednisolone remains obscure, although in part it is due to an effect on the inflammatory response and white cell function. There is no evidence that prednisolone acts to inhibit prostaglandin synthetase activity. Prednisone itself is metabolized in the liver to the active drug form, prednisolone, but there is no evidence that more powerful anti-inflammatory agents such as betamethasone offer any advantages over these drugs, since the list of side-effects is correspondingly increased. Corticosteroid therapy is relatively contraindicated in a number of conditions including peptic ulcer, hypertension, and congestive cardiac failure, all of which may be exacerbated by steroid therapy. Corticosteroid therapy is, of course, indicated in a wide variety of medical conditions including idiopathic thrombocytopenia and exfoliative dermatitis.

A 43-year-old housewife complains of feeling profoundly depressed. She has been waking early in the morning, weeping frequently, and for more than two weeks she has been unable to bring herself to leave her home.

209.1 **The following drugs could be responsible:**
(a) Propranolol.
(b) Indomethacin.
(c) Methyldopa.
(d) Dextropropoxyphene.
(e) Cimetidine.

209.2 **The following treatments are likely to be appropriate first choices for this patient:**
(a) Chlorpromazine.
(b) Mianserin.
(c) Diazepam.
(d) Amantidine.
(e) Lithium carbonate.

209.3 **She is referred to a psychiatrist who recommends the tricyclic antidepressant amitriptyline:**
(a) Improvement in depressive symptoms should occur within 24–48 hours.
(b) Dry mouth is a frequent side-effect.
(c) This class of drug is most effective if continued as lifelong therapy.
(d) It is advantageously administered at night because it has a mild sedative effect.
(e) Diabetes insipidus is a rare but important side-effect.

209.4 **After several years of further psychiatric problems it becomes clear that this woman suffers from a severe bipolar depressive illness. Lithium therapy is considered:**
(a) Therapeutic drug level monitoring is required.
(b) Cerebellar disturbance is a manifestation of toxicity.
(c) Diuretics or low-salt diet may aggravate lithium toxicity.
(d) A Parkinsonian syndrome is common when high doses are given for a prolonged time.
(e) It is associated with the side-effect of diabetes insipidus.

209.1 (a) *False.*   **209.2** (a) *False.*   **209.3** (a) *False.*   **209.4** (a) *True.*
    (b) *False.*   (b) *True.*   (b) *True.*   (b) *True.*
    (c) *True.*   (c) *False.*   (c) *False.*   (c) *True.*
    (d) *False.*   (d) *False.*   (d) *True.*   (d) *False.*
    (e) *False.*   (e) *False.*   (e) *False.*   (e) *True.*

While a general lassitude is a feature of long-term beta-blocker treatment, and hallucinations and nightmares may occur with propranolol (and other lipid-soluble beta-blockers), overt depression is not seen. Similarly, CNS side-effects occur with indomethacin (hallucinations and confusion, especially in the elderly) and dextropropoxyphene (mild euphoria), but not depression. Methyldopa can cause a clinically significant depressive illness, in addition to sedation, drowsiness and lethargy, although early wakening and tearfulness are not common features. Cimetidine ordinarily causes no neurological symptoms, but at toxic concentration (e.g. in renal dysfunction or in the elderly) can produce confusion and ataxia. These symptoms are suggestive of a genuine depressive illness requiring therapy, and the usual starting treatment is a tricyclic antidepressant such as amitriptyline or one of the alternative types of antidepressant such as the tetracyclic mianserin. Diazepam may be useful adjunctive therapy, but chlorpromazine would only be indicated if the illness was thought to represent a major psychosis, and similarly lithium carbonate would usually be preferred for bipolar depression. Amantadine was developed as an antiviral agent but is more frequently used as an antiparkinsonian drug. The tricyclic antidepressants are often complicated by mild sedative effects and therefore may be most conveniently administered at night. The anticholinergic effects are also frequent, typically producing a dry mouth, and in overdose this can be a particular problem with respect to tachycardia and the risk of convulsions. Improvement in symptoms is often delayed for one or two weeks and therapy seems to be most advantageously applied if it is administered in courses of several months and then withdrawn, to be reintroduced should the symptoms recur at a later date. Diabetes insipidus is a side-effect of lithium carbonate not of amitriptyline. The precise mechanisms of action of both tricyclic antidepressants and lithium remain obscure, but both are said to promote neurotransmitter release. Lithium additionally is thought to reduce the excitability of cell membranes. Adverse effects from lithium, which include nausea and vomiting, confusion and drowsiness, and cerebellar disturbance, are dose-related, and toxicity may be precipitated by disturbances in sodium and fluid balance.

A 26-year-old schoolteacher presents to her general practitioner with a 4-week history of thirst, polyuria and weight loss. He checks her urine for glucose and ketones, both of which are strongly positive. The patient, although overweight, has been previously well and her only medication is the combined oestrogen–progestogen oral contraceptive pill. The diagnosis of diabetic ketoacidosis is made.

210.1   The following management plans are appropriate:
   (a)   Commence treatment with metformin.
   (b)   Prescription of an antibiotic for a urinary tract infection and review in two weeks.
   (c)   Advise to stop the 'pill', lose weight and otherwise continue at home.
   (d)   Admission to hospital for fluid replacement and insulin therapy.
   (e)   Admission to hospital for treatment with a sulphonylurea.

210.2   If a diagnosis of diabetic ketoacidosis is confirmed, which of the following are recommended:
   (a)   Hourly doses of subcutaneous soluble insulin.
   (b)   Soluble insulin via an infusion pump.
   (c)   Lente insulin by repeated intravenous bolus injections.
   (d)   Several litres of sodium bicarbonate ($NaHCO_3$) to correct quickly the metabolic acidosis.
   (e)   Potassium supplementation.

210.3   It is decided that the 'pill' has been a precipitating factor in this woman's diabetes mellitus. The following other conditions are well-recognized complications of the use of the oral contraceptive agent:
   (a)   Jaundice.
   (b)   Hyperthyroidism.
   (c)   Migraine.
   (d)   Hypertension.
   (e)   Osteoporosis.

210.4   Other drugs may in future complicate the management of this patient with insulin-dependent diabetes:
   (a)   Bendrofluazide.
   (b)   Chlorpheniramine.
   (c)   Prednisolone.
   (d)   Propranolol.
   (e)   Indomethacin.

210.1 (a) *False.*   **210.2** (a) *True.*   **210.3** (a) *True.*   **210.4** (a) *True.*
       (b) *False.*   (b) *True.*   (b) *False.*   (b) *False.*
       (c) *False.*   (c) *False.*   (c) *True.*   (c) *True.*
       (d) *True.*   (d) *False.*   (d) *True.*   (d) *True.*
       (e) *False.*   (e) *True.*   (e) *False.*   (e) *False.*

The patient gives a convincing history suggestive of diabetes mellitus, and the presence of strongly positive ketonuria indicates the need for admission to hospital for fluid replacement and insulin therapy. Other measures, such as treatment with an oral hypoglycaemic agent, either metformin or a sulphonylurea, are inadequate, and similarly treatment of precipitating or complicating factors, such as the oral contraceptive agent or a urinary tract infection, are also inadequate at this stage. The treatment of diabetic ketoacidosis follows several litres of fluid replacement and the administration of insulin. Insulin should be administered in a short-acting form either by repeated subcutaneous doses of soluble insulin or intravenously via a low-dose infusion. While severe acidosis may require correction with small amounts of sodium bicarbonate the risks of precipitating severe hypokalaemia are a contraindication to the administration of large doses of sodium bicarbonate and the rapid correction of metabolic acidosis. Because there is a total body deficit of potassium (sometimes in the face of a relatively high serum potassium) regular potassium supplementation is usually indicated. The oral contraceptive agent is known to be a precipitating factor in the development of diabetes mellitus and similarly cholestatic jaundice, migraine and hypertension are well-recognized adverse effects. Hyperthyroidism amd osteoporosis are not recognized complications of the oral contraceptive. Similarly other drugs may complicate the management of diabetes mellitus, particularly bendrofluazide and prednisolone, which worsen glucose intolerance, but also the non-selective beta-blockers which affect the peripheral utilization of glucose and which may mask the adrenergic symptoms of hypoglycaemia. Diabetes mellitus is not a recognized complication of chlorpheniramine or indomethacin.

211.1 **Self-poisoning with drugs is one of the commonest reasons for admission to a general medical ward:**
(a) The majority of cases represent a real attempt to commit suicide.
(b) In more than half the cases a large quantity of alcohol will also have been taken.
(c) The mortality, despite hospital treatment, is about 50% of all types of self-poisoning.
(d) Benzodiazepines are the drugs most commonly taken.
(e) Methods of increasing drug elimination (e.g. forced diuresis and haemodialysis) should be used whenever possible, irrespective of which drug has been taken.

211.2 **In the treatment of the acutely poisoned, unconscious patient:**
(a) Cardiorespiratory support is of primary importance.
(b) Respiratory stimulation with drugs, e.g. nikethamide, should always be attempted before committing the patient to assisted ventilation.
(c) Gastric lavage is unlikely to recover more than 30% of ingested drug.
(d) A reliable estimate of the half-life of the drug can always be obtained from blood concentration measurements.
(e) Haemoperfusion dramatically increases the whole body clearance of any drug.

211.3 **Specific antidotes or antagonist therapies are routinely available for the following 'poisons':**
(a) Morphine.
(b) Paracetamol.
(c) Ferrous sulphate.
(d) Salicylates.
(e) Benzodiazepines.

211.4 **The following complications are well-recognized to occur with these particular drugs:**
(a) Supraventricular tachycardia with diazepam.
(b) Complete heart block with digoxin.
(c) Respiratory depression with salicylates.
(d) Pin-point pupils with amitriptyline.
(e) Acute liver failure with codeine phosphate.

211.1 (a) *False.*   **211.2** (a) *True.*   **211.3** (a) *True.*   **211.4** (a) *False.*
      (b) *True.*   (b) *False.*   (b) *True.*   (b) *True.*
      (c) *False.*   (c) *True.*   (c) *True.*   (c) *False.*
      (d) *True.*   (d) *False.*   (d) *False.*   (d) *False.*
      (e) *False.*   (e) *False.*   (e) *False.*   (e) *False.*

Self-poisoning with drugs is second only to acute cardiovascular events as a reason for emergency admission to a general medical ward. In most cases alcohol will also have been taken and the commonest drug group is the benzodiazepines. In the vast majority of cases it is not a genuine attempt to commit suicide, nor is it a manifestation of underlying serious psychiatric disturbance, and it typically reflects an impulsive reaction to a particular stress. With the emphasis on supportive management the mortality is less than 5%, and methods of active intervention, either to increase drug elimination or to stimulate the unconscious patient, should be avoided. When required, cardiorespiratory support is of primary importance and assisted ventilation should certainly not be secondary to the use of analeptic therapy. Recovery of ingested tablets by gastric lavage is poor with a few notable exceptions, such as salicylates, which appear to form a mass in the stomach, and anticholinergic drugs, which impair gastric emptying. Haemodialysis and haemoperfusion tend to clear the circulating volume of a particular drug, but as a general rule they do not significantly increase the total body clearance. While measurements of plasma drug levels are of importance it is not always possible to obtain a reliable estimate of clearance or half-life of the drug, either because of continued and delayed absorption or because of saturation of hepatic enzyme activity (zero-order kinetics).

There are a few specific therapies which are appropriate for the management of particular drug overdoses. For the respiratory depression due to opiate drugs, naloxone is a specific antagonist. The hepatic damage due to toxic metabolites of paracetamol can be reduced by the use of amino acid preparations, particularly those with an SH group, and in clinical practice N-acetylcysteine is preferred. The chelating agent, desferrioxamine, is useful in the management of ferrous sulphate poisoning. There are no specific antidotes available for either salicylates or benzodiazepines, although the former may respond to treatment with forced alkaline diuresis. Certain clinical features will reflect the drug's pharmacological activity; for example complete heart block with digoxin. Pupils are characteristically pin-point in opiate poisoning   and   large and   dilated   in   anticholinergic   poisoning,   such   as   occurs   with amitriptyline   and   other   tricyclic   antidepressants.   Supraventricular tachycardia is also a feature of tricyclic antidepressant poisoning. The metabolic   effects   of   salicylates   tend   to   induce   a   compensatory hyperventilation and respiratory stimulation, and both acute hepatic and acute renal failure may be induced by paracetamol but not by other simple analgesics such as codeine.

A 26-year-old man with chronic schizophrenia on long-term treatment with high-dose chlorpromazine, 500 mg four times daily, reports to the psychiatric clinic complaining of 'shakiness' of his hands. His only other therapy is nitrazepam as a hypnotic.

212.1 The following statements about chlorpromazine are correct:
(a) It has an alpha-adrenoceptor blocking effect and can thus give rise to postural hypotension.
(b) It has anticonvulsant properties.
(c) It has antiemetic properties.
(d) It blocks dopamine receptors.
(e) It increases insulin release.

212.2 On closer examination the patient is found to have cogwheel rigidity and hypokinesia:
(a) Drug-induced Parkinsonism is the likely diagnosis.
(b) Nitrazepam is a more likely cause of drug-induced Parkinsonism.
(c) Chlorpromazine induces Parkinsonism because of its anticholinergic properties.
(d) Phenothiazine-induced Parkinsonism is an idiosyncratic hypersensitivity reaction.
(e) Phenothiazine-induced Parkinsonism responds particularly readily to treatment with L-dopa.

212.3 The following are well-recognized side-effects of chlorpromazine:
(a) Alopecia.
(b) Hyperprolactinaemia and impotence.
(c) Hypothermia.
(d) Osteomalacia.
(e) Cholestatic jaundice.

212.4 A number of therapeutic options are possible in the treatment of this young man's Parkinsonism:
(a) Change treatment to depot flupenthixol which has much less likelihood of causing Parkinsonism.
(b) Change to haloperidol which is not associated with extrapyramidal side-effects.
(c) Add benztropine if the chlorpromazine treatment requires to be continued.
(d) Withdraw chlorpromazine.
(e) Change to amitryptiline which is as effective in the treatment of schizophrenia.

212.1 (a) *True.*   **212.2** (a) *True.*   **212.3** (a) *False.*   **212.4** (a) *False.*
    (b) *False.*   (b) *False.*   (b) *True.*   (b) *False.*
    (c) *True.*   (c) *False.*   (c) *True.*   (c) *True.*
    (d) *True.*   (d) *False.*   (d) *False.*   (d) *True.*
    (e) *False.*   (e) *False.*   (e) *True.*   (e) *False.*

Chlorpromazine is one of the phenothiazines and is a major tranquillizer. Chlorpromazine has a number of effects including weak peripheral alpha-blocking activity, antihistamine and antiemetic properties, and dopamine antagonist properties. It also has a tendency, particularly in overdosage, to precipitate convulsions and to induce hypothermia as a result of an action in the hypothalamus. It has no effect on insulin release or glucose metabolism. Drug-induced Parkinsonism is a relatively common finding with high-dose phenothiazine therapy, particularly in the younger age group, and this appears to be due to the dopamine antagonistic action. This is not a feature of minor tranquillizers such as nitrazepam or of the tricyclic antidepressants, but it is also seen with the butyrophenone group of drugs, particularly haloperidol. This type of drug-induced Parkinsonism responds best to the anticholinergic drugs, such as benztropine, and does not usually respond particularly readily to treatment with L-dopa. Ideally the chlorpromazine should be withdrawn, but if it requires to be continued then concomitant benztropine therapy is usually satisfactory. There is little value in switching to a long-acting type of phenothiazine, which is equally likely to produce this side-effect, and tricyclic antidepressants are of little value in the treatment of schizophrenia. The only common hypersensitivity reaction which occurs with chlorpromazine is a cholestatic jaundice. Features such as alopecia, bradycardia and osteomalacia are not features of phenothiazine poisoning.

The following questions examine basic clinical pharmacological concepts:

213.1 Drug clearance:
  (a) Only refers to elimination by the kidney.
  (b) Refers to the volume of plasma or blood which is completely cleared of drug in a defined period of time.
  (c) Cannot exceed the glomerular filtration rate.
  (d) May be influenced by reabsorption by the renal tubules.
  (e) In principle, clearance is a concept similar to creatinine clearance.

213.2 The enzymes involved in drug metabolism:
  (a) Are located exclusively in the liver.
  (b) Invariably cause the loss of a drug's pharmacological activity.
  (c) Are individually specific for particular drugs.
  (d) Frequently produce molecules with reduced water solubility.
  (e) Have their activities induced by paracetamol.

213.3 The following observations on loading doses and maintenance (steady-state) doses are correct:
  (a) A loading dose is given to achieve quickly the desired drug concentration in the body.
  (b) A loading dose is necessary for benzylpenicillin which has a half-life (t½) of 30 minutes.
  (c) The time to reach steady state is a function of t½.
  (d) With the continued dosing it takes about four or five t½s to reach steady state.
  (e) If a drug is given until a steady-state plasma concentration is achieved and the dose is then doubled, the new steady-state plasma concentration will usually be double the original level.

213.4 Bioavailability:
  (a) Is related to the area under the plasma concentration–time curve.
  (b) Is more than 100% when the drug is administered intravenously.
  (c) Is increased if there is marked first-pass metabolism in the liver.
  (d) Is influenced by the pharmaceutical formulation of the drug, particularly particle size.
  (e) Is often influenced by the concomitant administration of food.

213.1 (a) *False.*   **213.2** (a) *False.*   **213.3** (a) *True.*   **213.4** (a) *True.*
  (b) *True.*   (b) *False.*   (b) *False.*   (b) *False.*
  (c) *False.*   (c) *False.*   (c) *True.*   (c) *False.*
  (d) *True.*   (d) *False.*   (d) *True.*   (d) *True.*
  (e) *True.*   (e) *False.*   (e) *True.*   (e) *True.*

Drug clearance in the body refers to the volume of blood (plasma) which is completely cleared of drug in unit time and is analagous, in principle, to creatinine clearance which is expressed in ml/minute as a reflection of the amount of blood which is cleared of creatinine in unit time. However, the major organs of drug clearance are the liver and kidney, and consequently drug clearance is frequently more rapid than the glomerular filtration rate, either because of a hepatic component to the clearance or because of additional active processes in the kidney, most notably tubular secretion. When drugs are metabolized the liver is not necessarily involved exclusively in drug clearance, because some drugs are metabolized in the gut wall and lining. The enzymes which are involved are not specific for individual drugs. The basic process is typically to produce molecules with increased water solubility, such that they might then be eliminated from the body via the kidney. The process of drug metabolism does not invariably cause the loss of a drug's pharmacological activity. The enzymes which are involved in hepatic metabolism may have their activities induced by drugs such as phenytoin or rifampicin (enzyme inducers) or inhibited by a drug such as cimetidine. With respect to dosing schedules a loading dose is typically given when the drug has a large volume of distribution, with tissue stores which require to be 'saturated' before the desired concentrations will be achieved. The need for a loading dose is not influenced by the drug's half-life, but it typically takes approximately four or five times the half-life before steady-state blood concentrations will be achieved, and at steady state the drug concentrations are usually directly proportional to the doses administered. There are notable exceptions to this rule, particularly phenytoin, which can more than double its blood levels when the dose is doubled if the state of zero-order kinetics has been attained, i.e. as a result of enzyme saturation. Bioavailability is the term applied to the ratio of the area under the plasma concentration–time curve following oral administration to the AUC following intravenous administration, with the latter being taken as 100%. If there is marked first-pass metabolism following oral administration then relatively little of the total amount of drug taken by mouth will reach the systemic circulation and consequently the bioavailability will be low. Similarly, if absorption from the GI tract is impaired as a result of the presence of food in the GI tract, or as the result of the pharmaceutical formulation, then bioavailability will be reduced.

214.1 **A 30-year-old woman has an increased chance of a venous thromboembolic episode if she takes an oestrogen-containing oral contraceptive and additionally:**
  (a) Is a heavy smoker.
  (b) Suffers from obesity and gallbladder disease.
  (c) Has had a previous deep venous thrombosis.
  (d) Uses a 'pill' which also contains a progestogen dose in excess of 50 μg.
  (e) Receives rifampicin and isoniazid, for treatment of pulmonary TB.

214.2 **The efficacy of her oral contraceptive is likely to be impaired:**
  (a) By the concurrent administration of phenytoin.
  (b) By the concurrent administration of cimetidine.
  (c) If she develops a urinary tract infection.
  (d) As she grows older, particularly over the age of 40 years.
  (e) If she requires corticosteroid therapy for asthma.

214.3 **Oestrogen-containing oral contraceptive drugs are not free of side-effects. Which of the following are true of oral contraceptive drugs?**
  (a) Migraine is likely to be worsened.
  (b) Should be avoided by women who are breast-feeding.
  (c) Hyperthyroidism may be precipitated.
  (d) There is an increased incidence of ovarian tumours.
  (e) Cholestatic jaundice is a recognized side-effect.

214.4 **This patient unfortunately develops asthma which is difficult to control with bronchodilator therapy and she requires oral prednisolone, initially in a dose of 20 mg four times daily.**
  (a) A total daily dose of 40 mg prednisolone is comparable to physiological levels of corticosteroid.
  (b) With low doses of corticosteroids, it is preferable to simulate circadian rhythm by administering 2/3 dose in the morning and 1/3 in the evening.
  (c) With high doses of corticosteroids, adverse effects invariably occur, even after a few months' treatment.
  (d) Suppression of the function of the adrenal gland, and therefore risk of acute adrenal insufficiency, is a recognized hazard of long-term steroid therapy.
  (e) Prednisolone is the most commonly used mineralocorticoid type of steroid.

214.1 (a) *False.*   **214.2** (a) *True.*   **214.3** (a) *True.*   **214.4** (a) *False.*
     (b) *False.*   (b) *False.*   (b) *False.*   (b) *True.*
     (c) *True.*   (c) *False.*   (c) *False.*   (c) *True.*
     (d) *False.*   (d) *False.*   (d) *False.*   (d) *True.*
     (e) *False.*   (e) *True.*   (e) *True.*   (e) *False.*

The use of the oral contraceptives is associated with an increased risk of thromboembolic disease. This has been related to the oestrogen component, particularly if its dosage exceeds 50 μg daily, but the risk is further enhanced in women who have a past history of venous thrombotic events, but not in those who are heavy smokers or who are overweight, which increase the risk of myocardial infarction and stroke. There is no recognized association related to the progestogen component. Drugs with enzyme-inducing activity may impair the efficacy of the oral contraceptive by increasing metabolism of the hormonal constituents. The converse is true of cimetidine which impairs hepatic enzyme activity. Similarly, efficacy may be impaired if there is concomitant treatment with another steroid which competes for a common hepatic metabolic pathway. There is considerable controversy over the question of antibiotic-induced 'pill failure', which has been attributed to changes in the normal gut flora and disturbance of enterohepatic recirculation. There is no evidence, however, that infection, or age, *per se* will influence the efficacy.

Cholestatic jaundice is a well-recognized side-effect, and both migraine and hypertension in the previous history should be taken as relative contraindications to this treatment. There is no conclusive evidence of an increased incidence of carcinoma and there are no obvious adverse effects upon the breast-feeding infant.

Apart from the combined-hormone oral contraceptives prednisolone is the most commonly prescribed steroid. As with all anti-inflammatory corticosteroids it has pronounced glucocorticoid effects and is relatively free of mineralocorticoid actions. However, the mineralocorticoid component is sufficient to produce sodium and fluid retention, particularly if large doses are employed. The physiological equivalent for prednisolone is 7·5 mg daily as 5 mg *mane* and 2·5 mg *nocte* to simulate the normal circadian rhythm. Doses above the equivalent of 7·5 mg prednisolone daily give rise to long-term adverse effects and with doses above 15–20 mg daily these adverse effects will occur within 12 months. Adverse effects include osteoporosis, hypertension and fluid retention, susceptibility to infection, glucose intolerance, and classical Cushinoid facies, but the most serious is adrenal suppression. As a result of administration of exogenous corticosteroid there is no ACTH stimulus to the adrenal gland, which atrophies. Thus, in times of increased stress, when normally there would be increased natural production of corticosteroid, the adrenal gland is unable to respond and acute adrenal insufficiency develops. This condition is potentially fatal.

A shopkeeper, aged 61 years, consults his GP with chest pain and gives a classical account of angina of effort.

215.1 Which of the following options do you consider appropriate?
(a) General advice about smoking, weight, exercise, etc.
(b) Treatment with digoxin to prevent cardiac failure.
(c) Immediate referral to the coronary care unit.
(d) Sublingual glyceryl trinitrate to be taken as required.
(e) Hydralazine to reduce cardiac workload.

215.2 Despite following the initial advice and treatment, he continues to have angina of effort. Prophylactic antianginal therapy is considered and his doctor recommends a calcium antagonist drug:
(a) Diltiazem is a reasonable choice.
(b) Headache is a well-recognized side-effect of nifedipine.
(c) Hypokalaemia is a side-effect of all calcium antagonists.
(d) In practice, nifedipine and verapamil have comparable antianginal efficacy and similar antidysrhythmic activity.
(e) Constipation is a recognized side-effect of verapamil.

215.3 He is eventually established on routine therapy with a combination of nifedipine and metoprolol.
(a) Metoprolol is a cardioselective beta-adrenoceptor antagonist.
(b) A beta-blocker and a calcium antagonist have a therapeutically useful additive antianginal effect.
(c) Both metoprolol and nifedipine undergo extensive first-pass hepatic metabolism following oral administration.
(d) Both metoprolol and nifedipine have long half-lives so once-daily oral dosing lasts for at least 24 hours.
(e) Nifedipine is contraindicated in peripheral vascular disease.

215.4 He remains stable with only occasional anginal attacks while receiving nifedipine and metoprolol. At age 67 years his angina worsens until he is experiencing chest pain at rest. He is referred to hospital. Which of the following proposals are correct?
(a) Coronary artery dilatation is desirable and oral isosorbide dinitrate should be prescribed for this purpose.
(b) Organic nitrates act mainly by reducing the workload of the heart on exertion and therefore have no place in the management of angina at rest.
(c) The efficiency of the heart should be improved, and symptoms thereby relieved, with intravenous dobutamine.
(d) The combination of isosorbide dinitrate with nifedipine is contraindicated.
(e) Headache may limit the dosage of isosorbide dinitrate acceptable to the patient.

215.1 (a) *True.*   **215.2** (a) *True.*   **215.3** (a) *True.*   **215.4** (a) *False.*
      (b) *False.*   (b) *True.*   (b) *True.*   (b) *False.*
      (c) *False.*   (c) *False.*   (c) *True.*   (c) *False.*
      (d) *True.*   (d) *False.*   (d) *False.*   (d) *False.*
      (e) *False.*   (e) *True.*   (e) *False.*   (e) *True.*

Classical angina first develops on exertion. It is stable if the level of exercise required to precipitate an event does not deteriorate rapidly. It is usually treated with sublingual glyceryl trinitrate as required. Hospitalization is not usually required, although a period of rest and observation would not be inappropriate. There are no grounds for treatment with conventional vasodilator/antihypertensive therapy or digoxin. Beta-adrenoceptor antagonists have an established role in treatment: all are comparably effective, but the cardioselective drugs (atenolol, metoprolol) are often preferred. As an alternative the calcium antagonist drugs have recently assumed a place, particularly where beta-blockers are relatively contraindicated. There is good evidence of efficacy when these drugs are administered in combination with a beta-blocker but, because both verapamil and beta-blockers have negative effects on cardiac function, this particular combination is not recommended. Calcium antagonists are not free of side-effects, although these appear to be relatively few with diltiazem. The introduction of nifedipine is often associated with 'vasodilator' side-effects — headache, flushing, tachycardia and palpitations. In the longer term, ankle swelling which is only partially responsive to diuretic therapy has been noted. Verapamil has fewer obvious 'vasodilator' side-effects, but instead has negative effects on cardiac conduction which form the basis of its antidysrhythmic properties. Nifedipine has no clinically useful antidysrhythmic activity. Constipation is a feature of continued treatment with verapamil but none of the calcium antagonists has demonstrated adverse metabolic effects (on glucose, lipids, etc.).

When angina is precipitated by progressively less exertion, if this deterioration occurs over a short period of time (days) or when it can develop at rest, then it is said to be unstable and additional medical therapy is indicated. In this circumstance the patient is most appropriately managed in hospital when intravenous therapy with organic nitrates is often added. The primary action appears to be reduction in the workload of the heart but there may additionally be an effect upon coronary arteries to cause their dilatation. This latter effect can be demonstrated with direct administration into the coronary artery, but is not observed in the course of oral treatment. As a manifestation of its vasodilator properties, headache is a frequent early dose-limiting side-effect. The specific role of beta-blockers in unstable angina is controversial but certainly not on the basis of their causing tachycardia, for which they would be particularly appropriate. There is no contraindication to combinations of nifedipine, isosorbide dinitrate and beta-blockers.

A 22-year-old woman has had epilepsy for six years, and is currently receiving quite low doses of both phenytoin and sodium valproate. She has had no seizure for over two years. She attends her family doctor for a pregnancy test which is positive. She is about 12 weeks gestation.

216.1 The following are true about anticonvulsant drugs:
    (a) Phenytoin is the only anticonvulsant which is teratogenic.
    (b) Phenytoin and sodium valproate in combination are likely to be more teratogenic than either alone.
    (c) Both drugs should be stopped immediately in this patient.
    (d) A serum folate analysis is helpful in identifying teratogenic risk.
    (e) Ultrasonal examination of the fetus at 18–20 weeks is likely to identify major abnormalities.

216.2 The patient is changed to carbamazepine:
    (a) This is logical.
    (b) There is risk of carbamazepine toxicity unless the dose is reduced because the free fraction of drug increases with increasing gestation.
    (c) Use of carbamazepine means penicillin antibiotics should be avoided.
    (d) Vitamin K should be given to the baby if carbamazepine is given to the mother.
    (e) Carbamazepine is safe in breast-feeding.

216.3 At 38 weeks gestation the patient develops a urinary tract infection with dysuria:
    (a) Aspirin would be a suitable analgesic.
    (b) Ampicillin would be an appropriate antibiotic.
    (c) Sulphonamides undergo extensive metabolism in the placenta.
    (d) There is an adverse phenytoin – co-trimoxazole interaction.
    (e) Cephalosporins should not be given to a breast-feeding woman.

216.4 In the first post-natal week this patient develops a deep venous thrombosis and pulmonary embolism:
    (a) Warfarin should not be given to a breast-feeding woman.
    (b) Ampicillin potentiates the action of warfarin.
    (c) Phenytoin increases the risk of thromboembolism.
    (d) Anticoagulant prophylaxis would be advisable throughout any subsequent pregnancy.
    (e) Warfarin is a teratogen.

216.1 (a) *False.*   **216.2** (a) *False.*   **216.3** (a) *False.*   **216.4** (a) *False.*
     (b) *True.*   (b) *False.*   (b) *True.*   (b) *True.*
     (c) *False.*   (c) *False.*   (c) *False.*   (c) *False.*
     (d) *False.*   (d) *False.*   (d) *True.*   (d) *False.*
     (e) *True.*   (e) *True.*   (e) *False.*   (e) *True.*

All anticonvulsants which have been extensively studied in human pregnancy appear to be teratogenic, although the incidence of malformation is around 6%. Cleft palate, congenital heart disease and neural tube defect are the most common problems. There is evidence that drug combinations have a multiplicative effect on teratogenic risk. If a woman of child-bearing age requires anticonvulsant therapy, the aim should be to optimize treatment with a single agent, the choice of drug being determined by efficiency rather than teratogenic risk. Since the period of teratogenic risk is during organogenesis (around 18–55 days) it is illogical to stop therapy or to change to another drug at 12 weeks. Also, anticonvulsant therapy should never be discontinued abruptly. Although a low serum folate has been implicated in causing fetal malformation in general, and phenytoin causes a low serum folate, there appears to be no single relationship between serum folate and anticonvulsant-related teratogenesis. Ultrasound examination at 18–20 weeks will identify major fetal malformations. Anticonvulsant plasma concentrations usually fall during pregnancy, often becoming substantially sub-therapeutic. Progressive increases in dose are usually necessary. Since serum albumin falls during pregnancy, and the free fraction of drug therefore increases, it is appropriate to try and keep total drug levels in the bottom third of the therapeutic range. There is no carbamazepine–penicillin interaction. Vitamin K should be given at the time of delivery if women have received phenytoin, which lowers vitamin K levels, but is unnecessary with other anticonvulsants. Carbamazepine can safely be used in breast-feeding women. Aspirin, and other prostaglandin synthetase inhibitors, should be avoided at the end of pregnancy because of the risk of premature closure of the ductus arteriosus and of haemostatic problems in the neonate. Sulphonamides cross the placenta without metabolism and can, at least theoretically, cause kernicterus in the neonate. The sulphonamide component of co-trimoxazole inhibits phenytoin metabolism. Cephalosporins are safe in breast-feeding women, as is warfarin. Ampicillin potentiates the effect of warfarin, probably by destroying gut bacteria and reducing vitamin K absorption. Phenytoin does not increase the risk of thrombosis. It would not be necessary to use anticoagulant prophylaxis during any subsequent pregnancy, but prophylaxis would be appropriate during delivery and in the puerperium, when women are at greatly increased risk of thrombosis. Warfarin is teratogenic.

A 19-year-old university student with classical migraine for many years has noticed an increased frequency of her attacks during the preceding four months. She describes a typical disturbance of vision with a fortification spectrum followed by a left-sided headache which persists for several hours and is usually associated with nausea and vomiting.

217.1 **Which of the following drugs are known to precipitate or exacerbate migraine?**
  (a) The oral contraceptive.
  (b) Diazepam.
  (c) Tyramine-containing foods.
  (d) Hydralazine.
  (e) Propranolol.

217.2 **The following therapies may be usefully employed to control an acute episode of migraine:**
  (a) Combinations of a simple analgesic, such as aspirin or paracetamol, with an antiemetic such as metaclopramide.
  (b) Methysergide orally.
  (c) Ergotamine by inhalation.
  (d) Indomethacin by rectal administration.
  (e) Bed rest in a quiet, darkened room.

217.3 **Although her episodes of migraine can be quickly terminated with simple analgesic therapy, she finds that episodes are occurring sufficiently frequently to disturb her university studies and she requests prophylactic treatment. The family doctor decides to commence treatment with pizotifen:**
  (a) Pizotifen is a serotonin antagonist.
  (b) Lightheadedness and dizziness are recognized side-effects.
  (c) It may cause retroperitoneal fibrosis with long-term usage.
  (d) It is a powerful vasoconstrictor.
  (e) It can only be taken parenterally.

217.4 **She does not respond particularly well to pizotifen and a number of alternative therapies are considered. Which of the following are potentially useful?**
  (a) Propranolol.
  (b) Clonidine.
  (c) Prazosin.
  (d) Adrenaline.
  (e) Nifedipine.

217.1 (a) *True.*   **217.2** (a) *True.*   **217.3** (a) *True.*   **217.4** (a) *True.*
     (b) *False.*   (b) *False.*   (b) *True.*   (b) *True.*
     (c) *True.*   (c) *True.*   (c) *False.*   (c) *False.*
     (d) *True.*   (d) *False.*   (d) *True.*   (d) *False.*
     (e) *False.*   (e) *True.*   (e) *False.*   (e) *True.*

Migraine is frequently worsened by the use of the oral contraceptive agent and precipitation of migraine in this circumstance is a relative contraindication to its use. Tyramine-containing foods such as cheese and red wine are recognized precipitants in some individuals and the vasodilator group of drugs is also recognized to exacerbate migraine. In the management of an isolated acute episode quiet bed rest in a darkened room is often sufficient, particularly if a simple analgesic such as aspirin or paracetamol, with or without an antiemetic drug, is also taken. For more severe acute attacks ergotamine is useful therapy. Because vomiting is often a feature of a migrainous attack, routes other than the oral may be preferred. Indomethacin is not appropriate therapy for this condition. In the long-term prophylactic treatment for migraine the use of pizotifen is well established. It acts as a serotonin antagonist and has vasoconstrictor properties. It is taken orally and is relatively free of side-effects, although drowsiness does occur and other CNS disturbances are not uncommon. It is not associated with the long-term complication of retroperitoneal fibrosis which complicates the use of methysergide. For this reason methysergide is no longer used as the mainstay of prophylactic therapy but rather is reserved specifically for severe cases. A number of other therapies are employed with success in individuals and these particularly include propranolol and, more recently, the calcium antagonists. Low-dose clonidine and sedative/tranquillizer drugs, such as diazepam, are also used.

A 57-year-old woman with infective endocarditis develops progressive renal impairment while undergoing intravenous treatment with gentamicin and benzylpenicillin. Her only additional therapy is frusemide 80 mg daily. After six weeks of this therapy she has several grand mal seizures.

218.1 The following are appropriate steps:
  (a) Stop the gentamicin which is a recognized cause of seizures.
  (b) Stop the benzylpenicillin which is a recognized cause of seizures.
  (c) Stop the gentamicin because it may be worsening her renal impairment.
  (d) Introduce diazepam orally as prophylaxis against further seizures.
  (e) Increase the dose of frusemide since cerebral oedema is a likely cause of her epilepsy.

218.2 The following drugs are known to be largely excreted unchanged by the kidney and therefore may accumulate in renal impairment:
  (a) Cimetidine.
  (b) Digoxin.
  (c) Atenolol.
  (d) Hydralazine.
  (e) Lignocaine.

218.3 In this patient's case the gentamicin dose was adjusted in order to maintain therapeutic levels, and when the benzylpenicillin was stopped there was some improvement in the level of renal function. Toxicity attributable to gentamicin:
  (a) Can affect the eighth cranial nerve.
  (b) Is related to a duration of treatment greater than two weeks.
  (c) Is more likely if there is pre-existing renal damage.
  (d) Is more likely in the elderly.
  (e) Causes irreversible renal damage.

218.4 A number of drugs are implicated in causing renal damage. Which of the following drug and side-effect combinations are recognized?
  (a) Lupus erythematosus with hydralazine.
  (b) Nephrotic syndrome with penicillamine.
  (c) Acute tubular necrosis with digoxin.
  (d) Crystalluria with allopurinol.
  (e) Acute interstitial nephritis with penicillin.

218.1 (a) *False.*   **218.2** (a) *True.*   **218.3** (a) *True.*   **218.4** (a) *True.*
     (b) *True.*   (b) *True.*   (b) *False.*   (b) *True.*
     (c) *True.*   (c) *True.*   (c) *True.*   (c) *False.*
     (d) *False.*   (d) *False.*   (d) *True.*   (d) *False.*
     (e) *False.*   (e) *False.*   (e) *False.*   (e) *True.*

Penicillins are generally free of serious side-effects. However, when administered in high doses and in the presence of renal impairment benzylpenicillin may accumulate sufficiently to cause CNS toxic effects, including convulsions. This is not a recognized side-effect of gentamicin whose most frequent adverse effect is renal impairment. Toxicity from gentamicin typically manifests as either damage to the kidneys or as damage to the high-frequency auditory component of the eighth cranial nerve. Toxicity appears to be plasma concentration-related but it has not yet been clearly established whether it is high peak levels or sustained elevation of trough levels which are responsible. Duration of treatment *per se* is not a critical factor. Even allowing for the fact that gentamicin accumulation is more likely to occur in the presence of pre-existing renal impairment there is an increased susceptibility to renal damage in patients with pre-existing renal disease, in the elderly, in those exposed to hypovolaemia or hypotension, and arguably also in those concomitantly treated with frusemide and cephalosporins. The damage to the kidney at its most severe produces acute tubular necrosis and acute renal failure but typically there is a complete recovery with time. Renal damage and renal complications are also associated with drugs such as penicillamine and gold, which are used in the management of rheumatoid arthritis. These drugs give rise to proteinuria and the nephrotic syndrome. A drug-induced lupus erythematosus syndrome is associated with hydralazine, particularly in slow acetylators, and particularly with high doses administered for a long period. The drug-induced LE syndrome is also a complication of procainamide and isoniazid therapies. No significant renal impairment is associated with digoxin, but as a rare complication of penicillin therapy, especially methicillin, there may be acute interstitial nephritis which is a hypersensitivity reaction (delayed type). As allopurinol prevents the formation of uric acid it is not associated with the development of crystalluria. Aside from causing renal damage a number of drugs are excreted almost exclusively by the kidney and these may accumulate in renal failure. Such drugs include digoxin and atenolol, but cimetidine, hydralazine and lignocaine are all extensively metabolized in the liver.

Oral diazepam is not effective as prophylaxis against epilepsy.

A 24-year-old professional footballer attends his general practitioner complaining of three weeks of persistent epigastric discomfort, most marked two hours after eating and wakening him from sleep.

219.1 The following are appropriate initial recommendations:
  (a) Aspirin as required to relieve the discomfort.
  (b) A prescription for aluminium hydroxide and arrangements made for a barium meal.
  (c) Advice to stop smoking.
  (d) A course of metoclopramide to reduce gastric acidity.
  (e) A small regular dose of a tranquillizer, e.g. diazepam.

219.2 He is found to have a chronic duodenal ulcer on gastroscopy. Which of the following treatments are of proven benefit in healing duodenal ulcers?
  (a) Antacid therapy.
  (b) Carbenoxolone.
  (c) Sucralfate.
  (d) Ranitidine.
  (e) Metoclopramide.

219.3 He is given a four-week course of twice-daily cimetidine. The following are well-recognized side-effects of cimetidine:
  (a) Gynaecomastia.
  (b) Mental confusion, especially in elderly patients.
  (c) Fluid retention and potassium loss.
  (d) Constipation.
  (e) Systemic alkalosis.

219.4 Cimetidine is known to interact with other drugs giving rise to potentially adverse consequences:
  (a) This is due to its competing for protein binding sites.
  (b) It is a powerful enzyme inducer.
  (c) It may potentiate the effects of warfarin.
  (d) Dosage adjustment is likely to be required if the patient is receiving phenytoin.
  (e) Dosage adjustment is likely to be required if the patient is receiving gentamicin.

219.1 (a) *False.*　**219.2** (a) *True.*　**219.3** (a) *True.*　**219.4** (a) *False.*
　　　　(b) *True.*　　　　　(b) *True.*　　　　　(b) *True.*　　　　　(b) *False.*
　　　　(c) *True.*　　　　　(c) *True.*　　　　　(c) *False.*　　　　　(c) *True.*
　　　　(d) *False.*　　　　(d) *True.*　　　　　(d) *False.*　　　　　(d) *True.*
　　　　(e) *False.*　　　　(e) *False.*　　　　(e) *False.*　　　　(e) *False.*

Because of their well-recognized propensity for causing gastric side-effects, including gastric erosions, aspirin and other non-steroidal anti-inflammatory drugs are inappropriate for this type of pain. Cessation of smoking and bed rest are useful adjunctive therapies for ulcer healing, but there is no evidence that tranquillizer/sedative drugs have any useful role to play. Symptomatic relief is frequently obtained using small doses of aluminium hydroxide, and as this therapy has no serious side-effects it is useful symptomatic treatment while awaiting the results of further investigations. A number of therapies have been shown to improve the rate of ulcer healing and these include antacids, carbenoxolone, H_2-receptor antagonists, and sucralfate. Metoclopramide is not useful therapy in this circumstance and it has no effect on gastric acid output.

Although cimetidine is appropriate therapy for ulcer healing it is not free of side-effects. It gives rise to antiandrogenic effects, including gynaecomastia, and also can produce CNS effects, particularly in those with renal impairment and in the elderly. It does not have the problems of fluid retention and aldosterone-like effects which complicate the use of carbenoxolone, and similarly is not associated with any upset in bowel function, neither constipation, as with aluminium hydroxide, nor diarrhoea, as with magnesium trisilicate. Large doses of sodium bicarbonate, classically with large amounts of milk, are associated with systemic alkalosis because the bicarbonate component is absorbed from the GI tract.

The antiandrogenic side-effects of cimetidine are not shared by ranitidine, and similarly the effects on liver function appear to be peculiar to cimetidine. It acts to reduce liver blood flow and to inhibit hepatic enzyme activity, but it has no effect on protein binding sites. As it affects the liver's metabolic capacity it may potentiate the effects of warfarin therapy and similarly may interfere with the dosage of phenytoin. It should have no effect on the dose of a drug like gentamicin which is excreted by the kidney.

A 27-year-old mother of two attends her family doctor complaining of low backache and a burning sensation when she passes urine. A diagnosis of a urinary tract infection is made.

220.1   The following are appropriate steps:
(a)   It is essential to await a bacteriological report on a urine specimen before instituting treatment.
(b)   A prescription for oral ampicillin.
(c)   Referral to hospital for a course of intravenous gentamicin.
(d)   A prescription for an analgesic such as pethidine, which will not cause ureteric spasm.
(e)   Advice to increase her fluid intake and to take a five-day course of co-trimoxazole.

220.2   The patient is given a prescription for oral cephalexin. The possible disadvantages of this drug in this patient are:
(a)   It is eliminated primarily by the liver and so no active drug will reach the urine.
(b)   It is well-recognized to cause peripheral neuropathy.
(c)   It is a powerful hepatic enzyme inducer and may thus reduce the efficacy of the oral contraceptive.
(d)   Because it is potentially toxic for the central nervous system, ideally its blood levels should be carefully monitored.
(e)   It is only effective against Gram-positive organisms.

220.3   When she accepts the prescription for cephalexin she reminds her doctor that she is 'allergic' to penicillin:
(a)   This is of no consequence; patients allergic to penicillins have no greater likelihood of an allergic response to cephalosporins.
(b)   Cephalosporins and penicillins both have a beta-lactam bond as part of their structures.
(c)   Severe potentially fatal immediate hypersensitivity responses to penicillins occur in about 20% of patients.
(d)   Most penicillin 'allergies' are relatively mild, e.g. skin rash with ampicillin.
(e)   The skin rash associated with ampicillin is particularly likely if the patient's immune system is impaired, e.g. in glandular fever.

220.4   The woman returns, cured, two weeks later and says that she has fallen pregnant. Which of the following antimicrobial drugs are considered safe in early pregnancy?
(a)   Flucloxacillin.
(b)   Oxytetracycline.
(c)   Trimethoprim.
(d)   Gentamicin.
(e)   Cephalexin.

220.1 (a) *False.*   **220.2** (a) *False.*   **220.3** (a) *False.*   **220.4** (a) *True.*
    (b) *True.*   (b) *False.*   (b) *True.*   (b) *False.*
    (c) *False.*   (c) *False.*   (c) *False.*   (c) *False.*
    (d) *False.*   (d) *False.*   (d) *True.*   (d) *True.*
    (e) *True.*   (e) *False.*   (e) *True.*   (e) *True.*

This is a common problem, and because the usual organism is sensitive to standard antibiotic therapy, for example ampicillin or co-trimoxazole, there is no specific need to await a bacteriological report. Increased fluid intake is useful for symptomatic relief, as is alkalinization of the urine, but there is no need for opiate analgesics such as pethidine. Similarly the illness is of insufficient severity to warrant hospital referral. The cephalosporin group of antibacterial drugs are similar to the penicillins insofar as they have a beta-lactam ring as part of their structures. They are also subject to renal elimination both by glomerular filtration and by active renal tubular secretion and they have no effects on hepatic function. They are relatively free of side-effects and toxic effects and they have a broad spectrum of antibacterial activity. Rarely patients who are allergic to penicillins share a hypersensitivity response to cephalosporins. However, as severe hypersensitivity reactions to penicillins occur in less than 0·1% of patients this cross-sensitivity is of limited clinical relevance. In many cases patients who complain of being allergic to penicillin are referring to the common skin rash (20%) which occurs with ampicillin. This side-effect of ampicillin is not a genuine manifestation of penicillin allergy and is recognized to occur even more frequently if the patient's immune system is impaired; for example in glandular fever the incidence of skin rash is approximately 90%. In the course of pregnancy both the penicillins and the cephalosporins are considered to be safe, but drugs such as oxytetracycline (bone growth impairment) and trimethoprim (folate antagonist) should be avoided.